Breaking Free challenges conventional wisdom. In this world of growing uncertainty, argues Dr. Kardener, only by abandoning childhood perceptions of safety will we find fulfillment in our adult life. Easily accessible and distilled from 40 years of the author's experience as a front-line therapist and teacher, this book will be valuable to laymen and professionals alike.

Peter C. Whybrow, M.D. - Director, Semel Institute for Neuroscience and Human Behavior at UCLA. Author, *A Mood Apart: The Thinker's Guide to Emotion and Its Disorder.*

In this illuminating and original book, Dr. Sheldon Kardener, an experienced and wise practicing psychiatrist, synthesizes a wide range of developmental, psychological, interpersonal, and biological views on how we start out in life, how we evolve into sometime struggling adults, and how we might transcend and transform into healthier selves. Dr. Kardener's perspective, honed over decades of psychotherapy practice and teaching at UCLA and elsewhere, integrates a wide range of theories addressing how psychological difficulties emerge. With close attention to psychoanalytic, psychodynamic, existential, transactional, and spiritual traditions, his ideas offer pathways to attaining a better life through resolving old conflicts.

Joel Yager, M.D. - Professor of Psychiatry, School of Medicine, University of Colorado

In clear, non-technical language Dr. Kardener draws on his considerable psychiatric teaching and practice experience to illustrate not only how - *but especially why* - experiences as a child can seriously impact and impair later functioning and how as an adult desired goals may be restored and achieved.

Harold Gould - Five time Emmy award winning stage, screen, and television actor.

If you want to finally let go of your past, so you can live to the fullest in the present, this book will give you both the way and will to do it.

> Mark Goulston, M.D. - Author, *Get Out of Your Own Way.* One of Consumers' Research Council of America's Top Psychiatrists – 2004-2005

Sometimes the most direct path to enlightenment is the best. Dr. Kardener offers such a path in his new book. We all know someone who needs to learn the truth. And maybe they will, if we can just get them to read this book!

> Robert A. Schiller - Emmy winning comedy writer of many TV shows including *I Love Lucy*, *All In The Family*, and *Maude*. Recipient of the Lifetime of Excellence Award.

BREAKING FREE

HOW CHAINS FROM CHILDHOOD
KEEP US FROM WHAT WE WANT

SHELDON H. KARDENER, MD

and

MONIKA OLOFSSON KARDENER, MFT

———

New York

Breaking Free
How Chains From Childhood Keep Us From What We Want

ISBN 978-1-60037-645-0

Library of Congress Control Number: 2009928324

MORGAN · JAMES
THE ENTREPRENEURIAL PUBLISHER

Morgan James Publishing, LLC
1225 Franklin Ave., STE 325
Garden City, NY 11530-1693
Toll Free 800-485-4943
www.MorganJamesPublishing.com

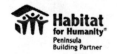

In an effort to support local communities, raise awareness and funds, Morgan James Publishing donates one percent of all book sales for the life of each book to Habitat for Humanity. Get involved today, visit **www.HelpHabitatForHumanity.org**.

Dedicated to

Gabriel and Aviva

the future

Contents

CHAPTER FOUR

CHAPTER FIVE

ACKNOWLEDGMENTS

My thanks to

All my teachers, who were patient with me.

All my patients, who were teachers to me.

My first professor of psychiatry, John Dorsey, MD, who taught me that, as human beings, we are all connected. We ignore this fact at our peril. This thought was conveyed in his first lecture, "My Beloved Nazi Physician." Now *there* was a talk that challenged me to be open enough to listen. Denying that each of us is capable of committing horrific acts, although we certainly may choose not to do so, is to deny the shared humanness we have with those who have chosen otherwise. Relegating those people to the category of subhuman is to choose to become one of them.

Louis Jolyn "Jolly" West, MD, past professor and chair of UCLA's Department of Psychiatry, researcher, civil rights activist long before it was acceptable, guide, friend, and—most of all—mensch.

Florence Bienenfeld, PhD, for her unflagging encouragement over many years to tackle the writing of this book.

Steve Price, PhD, for his friendship and his willingness to read the manuscript and give constructive feedback.

Lois Smith, without whose editing skills this might never have reached a readable level. Her encouragement, patience, and friendship are greatly appreciated.

Bill Gladstone of Waterside Productions, whose enthusiasm for this project was both enduring and endearing.

And most of all, to Monika, for her love, encouragement, exacting transcription of my lectures, intelligent comments, heated discussions, incredibly constructive criticism, and phenomenal rewriting and editing of the final draft. Although we have decided to retain the first-person-singular pronoun throughout the book, this does not diminish in the least the importance of Monika's collaboration.

INTRODUCTION

My desire to share ideas synthesized over forty years of teaching and practicing psychiatry motivated me to write this book. These ideas are meant to complement existing theories and to incorporate some of the new advances made in both the psychological and the neurophysiological realms.

When Neil Armstrong made his historic landing on the moon, the director of the National Institute of Mental Health said that perhaps we would soon be able to land a man on the surface of the mind as well. It seems the discoveries made in the field, and those that continue to be made at a dizzying pace, bring us ever closer to fulfilling that wish. Developments in genetics, immunology, neurophysiology, psychology, and biochemistry have illuminated the workings of the amazing physical plant we know as the brain. These findings make clear the interdependence of the brain and one of its major manifestations—the mind. We now know better than ever that the brain affects the mind and the mind affects the brain.[1]

Observational studies of mother-infant relationships, combined with the ability to image the living brain, have led to burgeoning growth in the knowledge of the brain's development and functioning, from earliest life to old age. Long gone is the Cartesian notion of a mind-body duality expressed as "nature versus nurture." It is now very clear that nature and nurture work in harmony.[2] The more we have come to understand that infants arrive with about half of their personalities "hard wired from the factory," the more—not less—important is nurture in molding and directing the child's potentials in the most advantageous fashion for both the individual and the society in which he or she lives.[3]

A recent study demonstrates that identical twins can differ in appearance and have different susceptibility to disease—referred to as *epigenetic modification.* These variations result from environmental influences that affect the way genes are turned on or off in each individual. As the twins age and are exposed to more environmental factors, the variations increase. Fifty-year-old twins have three times more differences than three-year-old twins.[4]

Research has also shown that the environment plays a crucial role in both forming the brain's actual structure and its evolution throughout life. The brain remains malleable and capable of continued regeneration and development. Evidence now exists that psychotherapy affects the brain's very structure and functioning.[5] Similarly, changing the brain, as with the use of medications, changes the mind. For example, depressive thoughts can be altered by psychotherapy, medications, or both.[6]

This book includes, in addition to my own thoughts, information I have synthesized from many other sources in order to foster an understanding of personality and conflict development and the ways we relate with one another. Both therapists and patients engaged in psychotherapy may benefit from these ideas. Recognizing the meaning of conflict expressed through symptoms can be a guide toward productive problem resolution.

Therapy is an adventure of discovery, growth, and change. I use the term *therapy* in the broad sense to mean not only the formal arrangement between a practitioner and a patient but also the idea of one's own personal growth. The terms *therapy* and *growth* have an overlapping concordance. Although I define therapy more formally to distinguish it as a very specific undertaking, its raison d'être is to support the individual's psychological growth. In this sense, therapy may be seen as a lifelong process—one of personal awareness, enhancement, and fulfillment—which may at times take place with a therapist.

I have tried to capture some of the old notions, the exciting new findings of the brain's plasticity, and the idea of growth throughout life with this couplet:

Geneticists have said you're done at conception,
the Freudians, that you're finished at five.
But let me tell you, brother, and let me tell you, sister,
you ain't done as long as you're alive!

This book's title, *Breaking Free,* conveys the essence of our human struggle in risking change. I introduce some preliminary core ideas in Chapters One, Two, and Three before describing the concept of breaking free. In the first chapter, I focus on the human infant's utter helplessness and his or her urgent necessity to bond with a caretaker in order to survive. This leads to the development of unique states of mind, which I refer to in Chapters Two and Three as those of **Child** and **Adult**. Though these words are commonly defined chronologically, the use of bold capital letters indicates that they refer not to age but to mental states. Each has its own set of characteristics, which will be described and defined.

After this introductory information, I present the meaning of *Breaking Free* in Chapter Four. How the shared ideas apply to our interactions with others—particularly in our marital choices and family relationships—is the subject of Chapter Five. As if rotating a faceted gem, I reflect on the enterprise of psychotherapy in Chapters Six and Seven. In Chapter Eight, I focus on three important concepts commonly encountered in psychotherapy before moving, in Chapter Nine, to clinical examples that illustrate the ideas presented in earlier chapters. Chapter Ten offers a summary of the core concepts.

To avoid the cumbersome use of "he/she" and "him/her," and to facilitate reading, I have generally employed the male pronoun. No gender bias is implied or intended.

Starting with the image on the cover, I have added visual representations to clarify the themes discussed, because images aid in the understanding of ideas and concepts by connecting thoughts (left brain) and feelings (right brain).[7]

CHAPTER ONE

In the Beginning

The human is born helpless. This is such a fundamental fact that we often lose sight of it. We are born developmentally premature compared with other mammals.[1] For example, at birth, three-quarters of the brains of our primate cousins is developed, whereas we start out with a modest one-quarter. The impact of this simple fact is profound.

In perhaps one of the greatest compromises ever negotiated between nature and evolution, we humans traded earlier independent functioning for larger heads to hold our incredibly complex and developing brains. Other mammals have a much greater ability to get going from birth or soon thereafter. As humans transitioned from quadrupedal to bipedal movement, the hips had to change to carry the greater upright weight thrust on the pelvis. This resulted in a narrowing of the birth canal at the same time that evolution gifted the human with a greater brain structure.

As the newborn's brain continues to develop and enlarge, he must utterly depend on a parent over a prolonged period. Although initially helpless, the infant is born with an amazing innate and vital capacity to capture adults' attention—a veritable repertoire of communication skills. Try walking past an infant without engaging his gaze, gestures, and smile. The invitation is harder to refuse with some infants than with others. Therefore, like any biologically determined element, this ability varies among infants, giving some a greater chance to connect with a caregiver, usually the mother.

1

Mothers also vary in their ability to bond with their babies. If an infant with low appeal is born to a mother who has less-than-optimal ability to bond, it portends trouble for the child. The vicissitudes of such difficulties in bonding are described in greater detail later in this chapter. The infant must, however, establish some kind of bond with his caretaker or he will literally die.

Think of how often an item in the newspaper or on the evening news calls attention to an abandoned infant found sometimes alive, more often not. Even with the new laws passed by some states whereby a newborn can be turned over to one of many authorities without any questions or legal repercussions, such stories continue to be reported. These stories of abandonment drive home the point that whatever the nature of the connection between the infant and his primary caretaker, it is always better for the child than not having any connection at all. We must accept whatever bond our parent provides us in order to survive. Furthermore, we must tenaciously cling to what we have if we are to continue to survive. If what we must cling to is destructive and impedes growth, a powerful conflict arises.

This imperative of bonding—a fact of life dictated by evolution—becomes the crucial nexus for the individual's healthy development and, at the same time, a major source of future struggles. James Masterson summed it up well when he said that three factors contribute to how our lives will turn out: nature, nurture, and fate.[2] Nature includes our genetic endowments, our deficits, and our own unique embryonic development and birth; nurture comprises the quality of our bonding as infants and the subsequent maternal, familial, and communal support available to us as we grow; and fate covers the uncontrollable vicissitudes that affect the lives of all of us. To have great genes and great parents but be run over by a truck illustrates the last point of fate. It is, however, these ubiquitous elements—our inherent helplessness as infants and our essential need to have some kind of bond to survive—that form the core thesis that I present in these pages.

Technologies and Theories

Advances in our understanding of what takes place in the developing human brain have come from many areas of research. Particularly important are the direct observational data from studying mother-infant interactions. Technological innovations have also provided the amazing ability to observe what actually happens in the living brain while the person engages in various tasks. Some of these innovations include PET, SPECT, fMRI, and MRI scans and enhanced EEGs.[3]

Along with these advances has come an evolution in psychoanalytic theory. Of particular importance is the development of object relations theory.[4] This theory led to a greater understanding of personality development and its dependence on the infant's interactions in his primary relationships as well as the subsequent recapitulation of these established interactive patterns with significant others in later relationships.

Early emotional experiences shape the brain, especially the right cortex, just as early physical injury in this area may show up later in life. Damage to the right hemisphere of a child's brain before sixteen months of age may manifest itself as abnormal moral behavior in adulthood.[5] The crucial role of this part of the brain will become more evident as I discuss the impact of the mother's mode of attachment to her infant.

The earliest psychoanalytic theories focused on the child's primary need to discharge his drives (mistranslated as "instincts" from Freud's use of the German word *trieben*). The role of the significant others in the child's life were viewed as secondary; their primary task was to socialize the child by providing acceptable ways for him to express sexuality and aggression. Children had to learn to manifest these primary drives in ways that society found tolerable.

Object relations theory changed this developmental model. While formulating object relations theory, professionals in the field, unfortunately, began to refer to the significant other as the *object*. Perhaps, in the future, the term *object* will be replaced with *significant other* or *vital one,* which more closely emphasizes the meaning of such an important relationship. Therefore, I prefer to use these latter terms instead of *object*.

In a previously published article, I noted that Freud was aware of the importance of the patient's relationships and that he urged therapists to pay close attention to their patients' familial circumstances.[6] However, the trend at the time was to focus on the one who had the symptoms. As a result, the vital ones were overlooked for a long time. Ronald Fairbairn, an early pioneer of object relations theory, cited Freud's paper "Mourning and Melancholia" as evidence that it was Freud who first brought attention to this new way of understanding how we attach to and then differentiate from our vital others. This deference to Freud does not diminish the significance of Fairbairn's originality of thought.[7] A schematic representation of the ideas contained in Freud's paper is shown in chapter eight, where I discuss the phenomenon of guilt.

Undoubtedly, as long as there have been Homo sapiens, parents have observed and been intrigued as well as puzzled by their children. But it was not until the middle of the eighteenth century that biographies of babies began to be published. Dietrich Tiedemann wrote the first known child biography, published in 1787.[8] Other reports followed by prominent fathers, such as Charles Darwin,[9] Alfred Binet,[10] and Jean Piaget.[11] With the development of psychoanalysis and psychological personality theories in the twentieth century came an increasing interest in observational studies of infants and, especially, of the mother-infant dyad.[12]

Only in recent years have researchers focused on the father's role. The dearth of prior studies may reflect an understandable bias, because the mother carries the fetus, gives birth to the infant, and nourishes the child. With the expanded view came the understanding that the father's involvement has a significant impact on the developing child as well. Infants whose fathers have been involved in their upbringing develop greater cognitive abilities.[13] Similarly, preschool children show superior verbal skills and a more secure mastery of their environment when dads take part in child rearing.[14] Other studies support the importance of the father's love in the prevention of delinquency and the development of self-esteem, superior academic performance, and psychological health.[15] Adolescents are more confident about themselves and their ability to deal with the world successfully when they have both parents' physical affection and support.[16]

Early theorists who promulgated the notion of the destructive "schizophrenogenic" mother soon developed greater empathy for her after meeting her husband and observing his behavior toward his wife. It is clear that mothers are far more effective in their ability to parent when their husbands are supportive of them and nurturing toward their children. If one thinks of a chair with only two legs as a metaphor for the mother-infant relationship, it is a far less steady structure, more easily disrupted by outside forces, than is a three-legged chair, the third leg representing the father's involvement. The more support the child receives, the better his physical as well as psychological development. Concerned with the ticking of their biological clocks, more single women make the difficult decision to have children through artificial insemination. It then becomes incumbent on them to have good support systems of family and/or friends.

Notwithstanding the awareness of the father's importance in rearing children, most researchers continue to focus on exploring the mother's role and her impact. A recent study reinforces the mother's primacy in her children's personality development. Eight of ten parental behavior factors that correlate with the likelihood that a child will develop personality disorders that arise in adulthood relate specifically to the mother.[17] Heinz Kohut is one theoretician who does include the father. In Kohut's terms, the father is a "second chance" for getting good parenting.[18] This presumes that the father is emotionally available and willing to counterbalance the impact of any unhealthy mothering. But the idea does not take into consideration that couples in conflict usually collude, which may limit the extent of the father's availability to the child. Couples' conflicted interactions often ensnare the children as well, for reasons that are more fully elaborated in chapter five in the discussion of how we go about selecting our mates. Common sense dictates that the father be recognized for his very specific and vital contributions to both his wife's ability to be a good mother and his children's mental health and potential productive roles in society.

Although researchers now examine father-infant interactions more often, my focus in this book is on the mother-infant relationship.

The accumulation of knowledge through research and psychotherapy has brought a greater appreciation for the intricacies of the matrix within which we grow and develop, especially as more studies about mother-infant interactions become available. As any parent with more than one child recognizes, the remarkable personality differences between children include varying abilities to capture the mother's attention, as attested to when one child becomes her favorite. All her children, however, must have her attention, receptivity, and caregiving.

The degree of fit, or attunement, between the mother and her infant not only assures the child's survival but also dictates the very development of his physical brain structure and whether he will realize his fullest potential. Recent findings have heightened awareness of the profound influence of mother-child transactions on the infant's brain and mind.[19]

The Impact of Deprivation

An infant without an emotional bond with a caretaker cannot survive. In the thirteenth century, King Frederick II of Sicily wanted to know what language humans would speak if they were allowed to develop that language on their own without hearing any other. Would it be an ancient language, a contemporary one, or that of the parents? He ordered nurses caring for a group of infants not to speak to them. Of course, prohibiting verbal engagement led the nurses to withdraw from all but essential physical care—there was no emotional interplay at all. The caretakers would otherwise have found it too difficult to maintain the silence and resist the seductive ability of the infants to capture their attention. What was the native tongue spoken by these children as they grew up? We will never know. They all died.[20]

Rene Spitz observed a similar outcome in his classic studies. A group of children reared in an immaculately clean nursery in an unnamed South American country were compared with a similar cohort of youngsters raised by their own prison-incarcerated mothers. The former group had clean clothing and bedding and good food but lacked any emotional connection. Sorely overloaded with work, the nurses had no time to play with, soothe, or cuddle their charges. They had only enough time to change, feed, and clean one infant before hurrying on to the next.

The prison-raised group had filthy surroundings, poor food, and more physical discomfort, but plenty of emotional connection with their own mothers and other women in the prison. In measuring and photographing these two groups, it became painfully evident how rapidly they had diverged in growth and development. The nursery group at each major stage—six, twelve, and eighteen months—were cachectic and underdeveloped; these children failed to thrive. The prison-raised kids were robust and healthy.[21]

A sickening contemporary example of this same phenomenon was brought into our homes via TV footage after the fall of the Soviet regime of children in Romanian and Russian orphanages who lacked bonding with any caring attendants. These children were profoundly stunted in every way. Carlson and Earls showed that these orphanage children had severe neurological and endocrinological abnormalities that may prove irreversible.[22] This kind of damage was also seen in monkeys raised in isolation. Nelson and Bloom demonstrated that these animals suffered disturbed behavior and neuroanatomical injury in the regions of the brain that are responsible for emotional regulation.[23]

Harry Harlow's early experiments proved how desperately infant monkeys needed to have "contact comfort." They would preferentially opt for terrycloth-covered wire forms of mothers rather than cold, bare wire surrogates. This is remarkable, because the bare-wired forms dispensed food. Both groups, however, showed severe damage, an inability to function in normal peer groups, difficulty mating, and, if they produced offspring, failure to nurture their infants.[24]

Good Enough Will Do

No connection means no survival. Does this mean that we must have a perfect connection in order to survive and thrive? No. That would require having perfect parents, and there are no perfect parents. Not only that, *there are no parents who were not once children themselves.* I will return to this point when discussing the impact of our unique familial experiences.

Donald Winnicott succinctly said that what we require is "good enough" parenting.[25] Such parenting allows the infant to connect for comfort and support and, when overwhelmed by stimulation, break the connection, then find that the mother is still there when he is ready to re-engage. It is crucial for the parent to remain available as the infant pulls away from stimulation and then returns. Mother must allow for and tolerate these disconnections and not thrust herself into that momentarily blank space. To do so would be for her sake and not the infant's.

The child is incapable of holding the image of the parent in mind—a phenomenon called *object constancy*—until about age twenty-two to thirty months.[26] Play a game of peek-a-boo with an infant, and you will see the apprehension on his face when you cover yours and then the exquisite joy of engagement when you show your face again. Winnicott beautifully summed this up by saying, "There is no infant without the mother." He commented that the infant finds himself in the reflection of the mother's eyes.[27] These statements are both poetic and factual. One cannot discuss an infant without the frame of reference of the dyadic interaction with the mother. This connection ensures the infant's survival and, with the appropriate attunement with mother, his thriving. The attunement takes place not only on a psychological level but on a biological one as well. It provides the fundamental schema for connecting with one's social environment in addition to that for internal emotional regulation. Allan Shore has shown that the infant's experience with his mother directly influences the development of his brain's physical structure.[28] Nature and nurture meet at this junction of the psychobiological connection between the mother and the infant.

As adults, we use such terms as "in tune with" or "tuned in to" in reference to our connections with and understanding of one another. It is this very essence of attunement that infants require and that we adults find so wonderful. Neuroanatomically, attunement involves the right orbital frontal cortex of the brain[29] which is the probable locus for the phenomenon of empathy, the profound connection between human beings. This is also the area where transference (feelings the patient has from past relationships, re-experienced in the present with the therapist) and countertransference (the therapist's past relationships re-emerging in relating to the patient) likely emanate. *Corrective emotional experiences,*[30] defined by Franz Alexander as important relationships relived without the associated prior trauma, may involve this same brain area as well. For example, a patient may experience the therapist as a supportive and encouraging parental figure, not the actual critical and condemning parent. By incorporating these new experiences, the patient may transcend the painful, old ones.

Some years ago, on the front page of the *Los Angeles Times,* I read about a fascinating, straightforward study. Unfortunately, I have not been able to find a reference in order to credit the authors. Because the work was so simple and elegant, I am going to mention it here anyway. The researchers asked a group of people if they had ever felt loved or been in love. Those who responded positively were then asked how they knew that what they felt was love. The experience called "love," they said, occurred when they felt understood or when they understood another person. This dramatically illustrates the powerful feeling created by attunement. We interfere with attunement when making judgments of others. In some societal situations, this may be perfectly appropriate, but an important caveat applies, particularly in emotionally intimate relationships: If we judge, we will likely not understand. If we understand, we will likely find little need to judge. This does not mean that we should overlook, excuse, or condone adverse behaviors; rather, we should focus on comprehending the *meaning* of the behavior.

Studying Infants and Mothers

The works of such pioneers in infant research as Stern, Ainsworth, Emde, Beeby, and Lachman, to mention a few, built on the foundation developed by Klein, Mahler, and especially Bowlby.[31] It is beyond the scope of this book to elaborate on their valuable contributions; some of the salient results will be mentioned in what follows. Suffice it to say that these pioneers' findings flowed from careful and elaborate observational studies of mothers and their babies.

Building on all these contributions has been the work of Shore and Siegel, who have explored the involvement of the mother's right brain as she expresses and processes emotional information, which serves as a master template for the development of the infant's physical brain structure.[32] I keep emphasizing the importance of appropriate attunement for the infant because with it, the mother imparts her capacity to soothe and comfort. When the mother offers a reliable connection, the infant can gradually develop his or her own capacity for self-soothing, self-comforting, and the ability to handle stress in the least debilitating fashion.

Mary Ainsworth standardized an observational technique—referred to as the *strange situation*—to categorize the ways in which attachments occur between mothers and their infants. A mother would briefly leave her twelve-month-old in a playroom with a stranger. The infant's reaction defined the nature of the connection with the mother. By Ainsworth's criteria, nearly 70 percent of American children have a secure attachment, meaning the infant becomes somewhat upset when his mother leaves but welcomes her return and allows her to soothe him. The initial rise in his stress hormones due to the separation soon subsides with the comfort provided by the mother.

Ainsworth divided insecure attachments into *avoidant, resistant,* and *disorganized/disoriented* subtypes. In the avoidant type, the mother did not display any emotional involvement with her baby when returning to the room. She seemed disinterested. The infant reciprocally showed no upset by the separation. He avoided the mother, focusing instead on toys, and moved away from her if she approached him.

The resistant infant experienced a mother who was disengaged by being emotionally preoccupied. This child alternatively showed clingy and resistant behaviors. When the mother returned to the room, he again focused on her but was unable to resume separate activities.

In the disorganized/disoriented group, the mother suffered from considerable mental illness herself. She may have been severely depressed, psychotic, or addicted to alcohol or drugs, leading to neglectful or abusive behaviors. In this case, the infant was unable to organize a response to the mother's return and actually engaged in self-harming actions such as hitting and kicking.[33]

Pruning the Neuronal Tree

At birth, the infant normally has an overabundance of nerve connections in the brain (neural synapses). A process referred to as *pruning*, selecting that which will be allowed to develop or atrophy, is necessary and natural to shape the brain's physical growth. An analogy is the evolutionary evidence that many now-extinct species once existed, but their lines simply disappeared at some point because they could not suitably adapt to or be nourished by the environment. The physical pruning of the brain's developmental lines follows a pattern referred to as *Hebb's law,* which states that neurons that fire together, wire together.[34] The old adage "use it or lose it" applies. This is especially true for the infant, but we now know that the brain remains plastic, or malleable, throughout our lives.[35]

However, even areas of the brain that are genetically determined to develop will be pruned if not used. Certain abilities we take for granted, in fact, depend on a temporal window. If stimulation does not take place during a certain period and the window closes, one loses the ability that would otherwise have been natural. Vision is an example. Hubel and Wiesel showed that if the appropriate part of the brain (occipital lobe) does not receive an image during infancy—say, due to corneal obstructions—the child remains blind even after later correction of that obstruction. The structures for vision, although intact, have atrophied in the meantime and can no longer serve their intended function.[36] Although this remains the common wisdom, very recent research demonstrates that the brain has a previously unknown ability to salvage some primitive level of visual function,[37] evidence of the awesomeness of neural plasticity.

All of the bad things perpetrated on a child can ultimately be categorized as either abuse or neglect.[38] When abused, the child is in a state of hyperarousal (from too much stimulation). An outpouring of the excitatory neurochemical glutamate occurs, which in high concentrations can be toxic to neurons. Some of the damage done to adult brains suffering from injury can also be attributable to the release of this agent.

In the case of neglect, the child suffers from hypoarousal (too little stimulation). This can damage an infant's brain through lack of necessary stimulation for neuronal development. Good parenting avoids both extremes of abuse and neglect.

Developmental arrest—disruptions of the normal evolution of psychological growth from infancy to childhood and beyond—can occur through either deprivation or overindulgence. The latter is a special kind of neglect, perhaps captured in the notion of "killing with kindness." The deprived child of the poor and the overindulged child of the rich may share the same misfortune of arrested development. If mothering is abusive, neglectful, or overly indulgent, the child's capacity to develop will diminish and he will be deprived of adequate defenses against stress. This has a profound impact not only psychologically but also physiologically throughout the person's lifetime.

Mary Main has studied the impact of insecure attachments on endocrine function.[39] The normal mechanisms necessary for survival, which enable us to handle acute stress and maintain bodily integrity, become exaggerated. Under chronic stress, the hypothalamic-pituitary-adrenal (HPA) axis and the sympathetic nervous system lose their sensitivity, and the system fails to shut off. Excessive pruning of neurons in the right orbital frontal cortex occurs. This part of the brain makes up one-third of the right cortex. Up to the age of three, the right hemisphere is the primary operating half of the brain.[40] The left cortex does not fully come "on line" until the fourth year of life.

The communication connection between the two halves of the brain, the corpus callosum, may suffer additional damage from stress, making it difficult for the right (emotional) hemisphere to communicate with or be contacted by the left (logical) hemisphere.[41] A T-shirt logo humorously reflected this by showing a picture of a frontal cross section of the brain with the statement, "Does your left brain know what your right brain is doing?" Too often the answer is no.

It is an awesome and sobering thought to consider that all parents—including those with unresolved emotional conflicts—in essence perform neurosurgery on their infants. They do so without a license and with training usually limited to what they themselves received as children. That the species survives and thrives is remarkable. However, this system of parenting requires more than just fine-tuning, as evidenced by descriptions in daily newscasts of people's inhumanity toward one another.

Numerous adult psychiatric disorders—such as depression, anxiety, panic, and posttraumatic stress—may arise from cortical damage.[42] If a parent's "broadcast" is not made on a soothing/comforting "frequency," the child may not develop a "receiver." Without a receiver, he cannot hear subsequent soothing or comforting messages from others. James Grotstein has discussed in great detail the profound impact in adulthood of a person's impaired capacity for self-soothing. Such an individual remains in a psychologically primitive state and cannot achieve internal emotional stability, which in turn leads to his having chaotic relationships with others.[43]

The severity of the abuse or neglect endured by a child determines the extent of the damage he will suffer, as well as the level of difficulty he will have later in life in repairing the damage. Hope ultimately rests in subsequent positive experiences of re-attunement with new, vital others. Certainly, a psychotherapist can play a crucial role. The fortunate individual will, at some point in his life, meet a significant person whose influence is both life-enhancing and therapeutic. The endeavor to repair, be it in therapy or through other relationships, is as worthy of the undertaking as it is fraught with difficulties. Nevertheless, the overwhelming emotional cost paid by the deprived individual throughout his life makes the effort compelling.

Connecting Is a Must

So crucial is our need to connect with a significant other that we will accept whatever connection we can get. For most of us, it is "good enough," but even if it is not, *it is always better than not having any connection at all; since without it, we cannot survive.* I continue to stress this obvious circumstance because the quality of the bonds we develop as infants and children determines whether our future will be healthy or troubled. The Dalai Lama was once asked to what he attributed his remarkable compassion. Was it to his Tibetan heritage, Buddhist upbringing, or perhaps reincarnation? He immediately replied, "My compassion and affection for all people, I learned from my mother. Please give your children maximum affection, maximum care."[44]

Think about the small child who has suddenly lost contact with his parent in some crowded public space, such as a fairground or a department store. That child might just as well be alone in the middle of a desert even though he may be surrounded by caring and concerned adults. Nothing—at least initially—will soothe him but the reappearance of his mother. If the child finally quiets down, he behaves like an automaton and exhibits limited emotional expression, in sharp contrast to his initial outpouring. The change to being quiet and compliant occurs when the child relinquishes any hope of his mother returning.

John Bowlby described three stages a child goes through in response to separation: *protest, hopelessness,* and *detachment.* At the loss of his mother, the child protests by crying, thrashing about, and resisting efforts to soothe him. After a while, if the mother is still absent, the child abandons hope, behavior that is characterized by whimpering, more passive withdrawal, and resistance to others. Still later, if the mother remains absent, the child enters the last stage of detachment. In this state, even if the mother does return, the child is unresponsive. He has disconnected and given up.[45] Unknowing caretakers often look favorably on this last stage. The child is now completely malleable and offers no resistance to ministrations. Understanding that this is actually a state of abject despair makes one less emotionally comfortable, since the ease of caregiving comes at such a high cost.

The nature of the attachment established with the mother dictates the child's response pattern. Those with secure attachments have greater resiliency.[46] Inevitably, when the child hurts, his natural tendency is to regress. This regression is either in response to the actual pain experienced or to the overwhelming anxiety of an event's anticipated unpleasantness. In the regressed state, children perceive comfort coming only from their mothers.

Adults of any age are certainly not immune to regressing. Comedians construct jokes around situations in which adults experience or anticipate fear or pain. For example, the reluctant astronaut who, when asked for his last-minute thoughts before liftoff, cries out pitifully, "Mommy!"

Those children with insecure attachments are further traumatized when turning to their mothers for comfort. The mother's inability to soothe leaves the regressed child with no alternative. He can only turn to mother, even if he senses that she is unable to soothe him. He may avoid contact, be resistant to it, or become chaotically disorganized when needing comfort. The absence of the mother's comforting compounds the child's original anguish.

When repeated instances of pain result in the child's experiencing more pain and no comfort, they become the paradigm for the future. Some people learn that they must pay a dollar for every nickel they get. It is not because they want such usury; they simply do not have any emotional alternative other than the loss of survival. If pain and distress characterize our primary relationships, we learn that distress *is* the cue that says, "I am home." No distress means no home. No home means no survival.

From this paradigm, it is extremely important to note that pain is never an end in itself. Rather, it permits a person to perceive and be reassured that a connection exists even if it is dysfunctional. People frequently continue to pay steep premiums in order to maintain old "life assurance" policies that expired long ago.

Jerry Kummer, a colleague, took part in a panel discussion on treatment options for teens on drugs. One of the panelists was a young man who was a recovered addict and successful peer group leader. In his enthusiasm about his program, the young man commented that he had never seen anyone who had been helped by psychotherapy. He suddenly became aware of Kummer's presence on the panel and blushed. In an embarrassed tone, he extended his apologies. My friend's low-key reply was prompt and to the point, "That's okay, I'd much rather be kicked than ignored!"[47]

In those words he summed up the core of the human dilemma. We are social animals, born physically helpless, who must bond to survive. We will take what we can get, even kicks. This observation correlates with research suggesting that being ignored is ultimately more harmful than being abused.[48]

Being Ignored Is Devastating

If a person believes that he must belong to a specific social system or group—just as the infant must connect with his mother—then exclusion from that group causes him agony, physiologically as well as psychologically. Imaging studies demonstrate that involuntary loss of connection to those perceived as important lights up the brain in exactly the same regions as does physical pain.[49] The response is even greater when judgments of shame, inferiority, or failure accompany the rejection. This makes good evolutionary sense, because we are social beings whose survival depends on social connections. Behaviors that might lead to exclusion from the group have to be avoided.

Susceptible kids who are excluded by their main peer group in school suffer intense pain. In the stunning incidents of school shootings starting with Columbine, the perpetrators violently visited their own distress onto the group majority. Through their actions, they tried to let the in-group know how much torment that group had caused them. They communicated their pain through *projective identification*—an action one person takes that results in the other person's experiencing what the first person is feeling. By making the other students victims, forced to face fear, pain, and even death, the perpetrators expressed their own desperate feelings. Unfortunately, this way of communicating generates a vicious cycle. Thought to be "weirdos" to begin with, the subsequent grotesque acts by those acting-out students only reinforced this perception, giving justification to many for having ostracized them in the first place. The vicious cycle closes on itself. Although this is an extreme example, people communicate their feelings through projective identification more commonly than we realize. In chapter eight, I will expand on this idea of how we let others know our feelings through our actions.

Exclusion from the group has been used as punishment throughout history. Ancient Grecians practiced ostracism for that purpose. More recently, the South African apartheid-oriented government used "banning" to negate the existence of certain persons. The banned ones could associate with only one other person, and nothing they said or wrote could be quoted or published. It was as if they did not exist. During the Cultural Revolution, the Chinese used ridicule, public humiliation, and shame to expel from their communities those deemed undesirable. In fact, the word *exile* is derived from *ex ilium*, which means "to be disemboweled"—a state inconsistent with survival.

These various penalizing mechanisms are not random in their application. Rather, they are calculated to revisit the infant's earliest primordial angst, the anguish of "no connection, no survival." This earliest, entirely real experience for the child remains as a remnant in every adult. Solitary prison confinement, no matter what rationale may dictate its employment, evokes the same profound anxiety.[50] That dread is what makes such imprisonment punitive. The painful threat of being returned to a primordial place of isolation enables others to gain control over susceptible individuals. Similarly, an exasperated or troubled mother may say, "If you don't behave, I'm calling the orphanage to pick you up." This elicits the same dread for the same purpose—to control the child.

The more intense our belief that we must be in a particular relationship or belong to a particular group, the more distress we feel if cut off from that group or relationship. In childhood, we learn which relationships and groups to consider important, and although our reality changes as we grow up, we retain those internalized cues. Intellectually, we may know that the very connections we deemed essential as children are destructive for us as adults and must be given up, but the earlier learned emotions may nonetheless powerfully contradict our relinquishing these connections. And so conflict results. This theme, conveyed by the book's title, *Breaking Free*, will be further explored in chapter four.

The Language of Connection

As I discussed earlier, it is impossible to parent perfectly. Besides, it would be undesirable. How would we ever learn to deal with frustrations if there were none? All that we require is "good enough" parenting. But that proves to be a commodity in limited supply—not because parents, other than those who are deliberately destructive and suffer from severe mental illness, willfully desire to deny children what they require to grow and thrive. Rather, it is because *we tend to parent the way we ourselves were parented.*

As infants and children, we learn and incorporate from our significant others' modeling how to relate in the world, and this forms our operating "software." Even if what we internalize is conflict-based and filled with error messages, we continue to use it until it becomes too painful. Only when we can no longer tolerate the pain, become aware of what we are doing, and realize change is possible can we develop new software programs. When reflecting on our own experiences with not-quite-good-enough parenting, we must step back and recognize that our parents, once children themselves, were also stuck with malfunctioning programs.

Research has shown that mothers' unresolved childhood conflicts greatly affect their ability to adequately parent their children.[51] Resolving these problems means that we must accept the impact of the limitations of our own parents on us. Understanding the nature of the childhood struggles of our parents helps us resolve our own difficulties more meaningfully and contributes to our no longer feeling stuck as childhood victims. After all, we are often the inheritors of unresolved conflict from many past generations. Gaining such a perspective allows us to empathize with and accept our own families. But most important, it allows us to accept ourselves.

The scripts we learn as children become deeply ingrained and difficult to recognize, yet they profoundly influence our behavior. Sigmund Freud's assertion that there are forces within us about which we have no conscious awareness that motivate and influence how we behave, react, and perceive our present reality contributed to the great resistance to his ideas by his contemporaries—and by many to this day. That was, and still is, a very large pill to contemplate swallowing. An anecdote told about Freud demonstrates the profundity of our unconscious scripts. Walking with Freud, an American patient voiced his uncertainty about whether to marry his fiancée. Freud responded that the decision had been made a long time ago, but that it might take a while in therapy to understand how and why.

Returning to King Frederick II for a moment, we actually do come equipped with a natural first language: the nonverbal language of the body and the musical tone of voice. Although usually only subliminally aware of it, we continually communicate through our body language. It requires only sixty milliseconds to read the emotions in a person's facial expressions.[52] This rapid subliminal awareness becomes conscious only sometime later, if at all. For this reason, the first answers that come to mind on multiple-choice questions are often correct.

Hunches and intuitive responses similarly manifest this "unthought thinking"[53] reaction, which is a valuable adaptive survival mechanism. Early humans had to react quickly to potential dangers without wasting time thinking about how to respond. This response mechanism may go awry in more socialized settings, however, where it may be akin to shooting first and asking questions later. People who are too easily riled may avail themselves of many anger management techniques, one of the most common of which is the folk wisdom of counting to ten rather than just reacting with the more primitive, emotional, right-brain responses. If the thinking left brain is engaged, one might not become enraged.

Communication between people consists of 55 percent body language (posture, movements, positions, facial expressions, etc.), 38 percent tonal quality (harsh, soft, kind, friendly, angry, etc.), and only 7 percent actual verbal content.[54] I have often thought a Nobel Prize would be fitting for the person who could delineate the complete vocabulary of this nonverbal language, as it is so pervasive in all human interactions. People skilled at reading nonverbal cues perceive a much richer and more meaningful communication than perhaps the sender of the message intended. Often we receive such messages without being fully aware of the total impact they have on us and then respond without full awareness of how much we are saying nonverbally. For example, therapists who use audiotaped or, especially, videotaped sessions often find that patients are unaware of how they sound and look when interacting with others. Almost universally, people are taken aback when hearing or seeing themselves on tape. The extent to which their voice tone and body language add nuances to their words often surprises them.

Marshall McLuhan[55] observed that "the medium is the message"— body motion, voice tone, and words. One of the cardinal characteristics of individuals who suffer from autism is their inability to read the full meaning of communications. They do not comprehend what the nonverbal expressions represent and become "lost" in social intercourse, unable to receive or send the nuanced signals most people take for granted.

Reading between the lines of a communication may contribute to our experiencing a more complete message, but it can also lead to misperceptions and assumptions. If we are unaware that past relationship experiences influence our perceptions of present transactions, we may behave now as we once did, or wished we could have done, in those original interactions. Our past experiences influence all our communications with others to varying degrees—that is a given. The only relevant point is whether we are aware of it. In psychotherapy, as noted earlier in this chapter, this influence is called *transference* (patient to therapist) and *countertransference* (therapist to patient). It may be a completely nonverbal and subliminal phenomenon. However, it is crucial that we recognize it, especially when the misperceptions could have deleterious consequences. Shadows falling from the past can obscure or distort our ability to see others in the present. It is the light of awareness that dispels those shadows.

Once a relationship exists, it is impossible *not* to communicate. This potent observation is true even if we are silent. Silence then becomes the message. We cannot avoid sending messages via our body language. The aphorism "You don't get a second chance to make a first impression" expresses the awareness of how much information we transmit beyond our words alone.

A study concluded with the observation that the therapist's evaluation of a new patient takes place in the first three minutes. (Frankly, I don't think it takes even that long). The remainder of the session is spent corroborating and confirming those first impressions.[56] The authors delineated the enormous amount of information conveyed through visual perception, body language, and tone of voice. Three minutes simply is not enough time to verbally convey sufficient content to reach the kind of impressions and conclusions that are drawn.

Another study, this one of communication between couples, found that it is possible to predict the viability of a marriage—whether it will ultimately end in divorce—by observing three minutes of interaction between the husband and the wife.[57] These powerful nonverbal communications are crucial in the process of mate selection, which is the topic of chapter five.

Memory

Considerable exciting research has questioned how we acquire, retain, and recall our earliest formative experiences. Until recently, memory was a mystery. Before we have developed language, we store our memories in the body. Daniel Siegel calls these *gut-level* recollections. They begin to form with the incorporation of the sensations in our primary relationships with our mothers—body awareness, emotions, and behavior—called *implicit memories*.[58] Such memories are not conscious recollections, and no verbal expressions are associated with them. Later we may subliminally re-experience those early memories in relationships with others in our first learned (nonverbal) language.

A vivid illustration of an adult in a deep hypnotic trance might make this phenomenon clearer. The man was asked to go back in time to his earliest traumatic experience. After just a moment, he began to shiver and gasp for air. He had no idea what was happening to him. Only later did he recall having been told that when a very small child, he had been thrown into a cold lake by an uncle. It was his body that had recorded and then recalled the event; the verbal memory came later from others.

Memories that we can recall verbally are referred to as *explicit memories*.[59] We begin to form explicit memories after age two and continue to develop them as the brain forms mature neuronal networks. Therefore, we cannot verbally recall incidents that happened before we were two years old. For most people, this normal childhood "amnesia" extends to the fifth or sixth year of life. Notwithstanding those individuals who claim to recall their transit through the birth canal, the neurological wiring has not yet been established to make such claims entirely plausible. The hippocampus, which is involved in forming memories, matures early in life; but early memories must be *stored* nonverbally, because the requisite higher-level cognitive functioning for long-term verbal storage and recall requires the involvement of the neocortex, which does not mature until the toddler or preschool years.

Memories from childhood are both reinforced and enhanced by stories told in the family about life events and by the child's gradually maturing skills, which also act to modify his recollections. An adult's memories of very early happenings—particularly abuse—require supplemental corroboration from others if such evidence is to be entered in any civil or criminal legal action. The whole danger of the so-called false memory syndrome must be avoided. In therapy, outside verification is ordinarily unnecessary, because the patient deals with his perceptions of what might have occurred and how those perceptions, whether factual or not, affected him as an individual. Who has not had the experience as a child of hearing someone say something that made a great impact but was of little note to the adult speaker? The heard message may be quite different from what the speaker intended, which is true of all communications, no matter what the ages of the participants.

The Narrative

The comprehensive story of how we understand our experiences—the narrative of our lives—is ultimately crucial if we are to resolve early conflicts and make sense of chaos. Societies achieve a sense of communal unity, identity, and history through their myths and legends. Similarly, the individual has to develop a cohesive story about his own life—one that explains the meaning of events that came to pass. Vital in the healing process, this narrative is required to be no more factual than a society's myths need be. Rather, it is the *comprehensive cohesiveness* of the story that counts—that it is well integrated and complete.[60] Consider the example of a deeply religious mother whose child has been killed. By understanding the tragedy as a manifestation of God's will, she may find solace and reach resolution. She then incorporates the event and its explanation into her life's story as comforting evidence of her conviction and faith.

The integrity—or lack of it—in our narratives will vary depending on the history of our connectedness, attunement, and security with our significant others. If our early relationships were less than optimal, we must as adults understand the reasons in order to form a comprehensive and healing narrative.

Having discussed the way we must bond to survive, and the impact our caretakers have on us both psychologically and physiologically as infants and small children, I move next to consider the characteristics of the **Child** and **Adult** states.

CHAPTER TWO

The Child and Adult States

Transactional analysis provides a clear, comprehensible technique for characterizing aspects of our experiences by describing the *Parent, Child,* and *Adult* states.[1] I gratefully acknowledge and deeply appreciate the clarity of Eric Berne's ideas. However, in this book, I modify his model considerably. I propose that there are only two states—the **Adult** and the **Child**—and subsume the Parent role into one or the other state depending on how healthily each functions. The enhancing aspect of the Parent guiding correct and appropriate behavior becomes the **Adult's,** while the restrictive, regressive components remain in the **Child.** When parenting is free of past conflicts, it represents a part of the **Adult** state that appropriately operates in the here and now. If unresolved childhood conflicts influence the parenting, it represents an aspect of the **Child** state.

In addition, I diverge from Berne's model by incorporating non-conflicted experiences from childhood—such as feeling joy, having fun, playing games, and solving problems—as part of the healthy **Adult.** Therefore, I use the term **Child** *only* when referring to *unresolved conflicts from past experiences that intrude in the present.* (It is the conflicted past— *still present*—that concerns and interests the therapist and forms the focus of psychotherapy. Issues that are resolved are truly past and usually do not arise at all, although they may be brought up as points of reference for success from which to draw strength. This will be discussed in greater detail in the chapters on psychotherapy.)

21

Each of us can appreciate having an **Adult** self as well as a **Child** self. Given that there are no perfect parents, it follows that there are no perfect adults. Some residual conflict from our childhood remains in all of us. It may not manifest itself until, or unless, we suffer some level of stress. Under sufficient stress—the degree varies from one person to another—all of us are susceptible to regressing or falling back into operating from positions of painful past perceptions. The coordinate system for the **Adult** is "here and now," for the **Child** it is "then and there." I believe that straightforwardly categorizing behaviors as arising from either the **Adult** or the **Child** aspects of a person helps to identify the origins of the behavior, assists in resolving conflicts, and thereby aids in the integration of the self.

Description and Characteristics of Each State

In every child (the actual individual), there is an emerging **Adult** (the state). As the child matures and has age- and ability-appropriate problems to solve and tasks to accomplish, the healthy **Adult** component of the self begins to develop. Requiring the child to carry out inappropriate tasks does not contribute to this growth. For example, asking a toddler to move a couch is an invitation for failure. Feelings of being overwhelmed and inadequate accompany those demands that are beyond the child's capacity. On the other hand, if the tasks and problems are beneath the child's ability, they are met with feelings of boredom, carelessness, and disinterest. In every adult (the actual individual), there remains residual unresolved conflicts—the **Child** (the state).

Below are the descriptions of the differences between the two states of being. The order follows that listed in the table.

Table of Adult and Child Characteristics

Characteristics	*Adult*	*Child*
Confirmation versus Validation	Desires confirmation from others but can only validate self.	Cannot validate self and must have others provide validation.
Analogue versus Binary Thinking	Analogue with abstract thinking capacity. Thoughts are not deeds.	Digital/binary with concrete thinking. Thoughts are the same as deeds.
Autonomy/Mature Dependence versus Immature Dependence	Autonomous and maturely dependent: able to stand on his own *and* be intimate. Engages in "love play."	Immaturely dependent. As a pseudo-adult, able to stand on his own while avoiding intimacy. Engages in "power play."
Vulnerable versus Helpless	Able to be vulnerable and no longer ever helpless.	Experiences vulnerability and helplessness as the same.
Choice/Competency/ Resources	Recognizes gaining a sense of these values as experiences accumulate and increase.	Is without, or unable to access, experiences that give these values meaning.
Alone versus Lonely	Can be alone but never feels lonely, as there is a sense of self as whole.	Feels lonely, as the sense of self is felt to be incomplete.
Empathy versus Sympathy	Is able to experience "empathy."	Capable only of "sympathy."
Desire versus Desperation	Motivated by desire.	Motivated by desperation.
Envy versus Jealousy	Can be envious and admiring of another's accomplishment.	Experiences distress, jealous of others' successes.
Wants versus Needs	Able to effect Wants even when counter to Needs.	Can only desperately hold onto perceived Needs.

Confirmation versus Validation

Because a child is helplessly dependent, he must rely on the vital others in his life to give him a sense of worth or validation. In contrast, adults can look only to themselves for validation of worth, value, confidence, esteem, and so on. In the child's life, those characteristics must come from significant others because the child's very sense of self is rudimentary and developing. (Remember, Winnicott said that the child finds himself in the reflection in his mother's eyes.) For the adult, others *confirm* but do not *confer* worth and value. It is a paradox of life that what we can get only from others when we are children can come only from ourselves when we are adults. This certainly does not imply that adults have no need for others. As a species, we are social beings who derive confirmation of our validity from good relationships.

If confirmation of the adult's value does not come from his relationships, he can do something about it. He can try to modify his interactions with those others, or he can choose new companions. But the child has no other options. Being deprived of validation leads the child to cling to the very source of deprivation—the withholding parent(s). He futilely hopes that somehow, someday, the vital one will come through. He will then have what he requires to feel empowered and will be able to move on. Without a sense of inner strength, moving on is as terrifying as jumping out of an airplane without a parachute. Further, imagine that the plane—representing childhood conflicts—crashed long ago, and somehow the child survived the crash and has grown into adulthood. It seems inconceivable that he would remain in the wreck of those conflicts, yet that is exactly what happens. To leave the crash site feels overwhelming; the child never heard the pilot say, "Go on! You're okay and can make it."

A scene from the classic film *The Wizard of Oz* beautifully depicts this idea. Dorothy and her friends the Scarecrow, the Cowardly Lion, and the Tin Man have struggled mightily to get to Oz so the wizard can give each of them what they so fervently want. In the midst of the wizard's phantasmagorical display, which holds the group in awe, Dorothy's dog Toto pulls the curtain aside, revealing an ordinary charlatan and not a wizard at all. They are crushed. All their hopes are dashed. Then the denouement: the wizard points out that what they have been seeking from him (validation) already exists, unappreciated, inside themselves. The only thing he can offer them is to confirm their validity.

It is not necessarily the actual parents to whom a deprived person clings. More often he holds onto the subsequent "stand-ins"—friends, lovers, and so on—whom he chooses specifically because they continue to prompt the same familiar deprivation cues that the parents provided. What a peculiar, powerful, and paradoxical state of affairs. *The less one got as a child, the more one clings as an adult to sources that perpetuate deprivation.*

The adult who operates as Child will stand starving in an emotional bread line waiting for the delivery of a crumb that tells him he has worth when right across the street there may well be a smorgasbord waiting. "But if I cross the street, I'll lose my place in line," he may rationalize. "When the delivery does come, I will miss out." This notion is captured in George Bernard Shaw's comment, "Hope triumphs over experience." (This statement satirically referred to second marriages).

Analogue versus Binary Thinking

A child's thinking develops through several stages as he matures. The toddler's mind operates on a digital, or binary, basis. This mode dictates all good or all bad, yes or no, up or down, black or white, all or none. It acts like a light switch that is either on or off. Piaget pointed out that between the ages of seven and eleven, the child enters the concrete operational stage and begins to develop logical thought processes. Through these processes, he acquires a sense of morality and awareness of self in the world. From eleven to the end of adolescence, analogue thinking and reasoning capacity evolve. This is the stage of *formal operations*, the age of reason when a dimmer switch replaces the light switch, providing an entire range of illumination between on and off. The growing capacity for abstract thinking can now supplant the child's concrete thoughts.[2]

Early on, if a small child fancies that he can fly, it becomes a fact to be tried out; thoughts and deeds synonymously blend. (With analogue capacity, the person can entertain thoughts knowing that they may be fanciful and not factual.) "Step on a crack and break your mother's back" is more than just a game, it is a way of preventing disturbing thoughts and feelings from translating into deeds during the stage of literal thinking. In a similar fashion, we use superstitions, a residual of this early mode of concrete thinking, to counter the fear that a positive thought will induce its exact negative opposite, unless we engage in a ritual to magically dispel such a possibility. "The medical tests were all good." (Oops, saying that means they could be all bad.) "Knock on wood." Saying, "It's a beautiful day for a picnic" might be met with the response, "Bite your tongue," no matter how blue the sky, as though such an action aborts the possibility of rain. Some people automatically go to great lengths to perform superstitious rituals based on this primitive thought process, frequently without any awareness of what they are doing or why.

This binary/digital mode of thinking, a natural stage of thought development, is inherently neither good nor bad but simply the way our minds work. However, the residual of this thought mode from childhood remains powerful in many adults. The power derives from both the absence of any alternative other than its opposite and the fear that thoughts equal deeds. (This is why Jimmy Carter's famous quote, "I have lusted in my heart," evoked fury among fundamentalists.) At the age at which a child's thought processes are functioning in the binary/digital mode, adults are teaching them what is right, acceptable, and proper or what will be judged wrong, rejected, and shunned. It can have great benefit or create great anguish as the child grows. St. Ignatius is credited with saying, "Give me a child until he is seven and I will give you the man."[3] Similarly, Proverbs 22:6 states, "Start a boy on the right road, and even in old age he will not leave it." However, when conflicts permeate what the child learns and remain unresolved in adulthood, this power fuels emotional distress. An adult who as a child learned to perceive himself as flawed may excessively strive for perfection in all his endeavors. He may hope the external results will, perforce, change the imperfect self-perception that drives his efforts—a mission impossible—as though it could be only one or the other with no middle ground. *The sculpture may be perfect, but the sculptor— never!*

Theoretically, every adult should be operating with analogue/abstract thinking. Sadly, this is not the case. Some 70 percent of the adult population operates in the residual Child mode with binary concrete thought processes.[4] Digital thought allows us to deal with the world's complexities in the easiest fashion. Reflect for a moment on the following examples, and you will recognize how very common, simple, and consequential binary thinking really is.

During World War II, and to some extent in the Korean conflict, Americans could see themselves as all good, dedicated to defeating the all-bad enemy. This simplistic way of thinking floundered on the rocks of the Vietnam War. The "enemy," Ho Chi Minh, declared that he admired Jefferson and the Declaration of Independence. Bad guys aren't supposed to do that!

Politicians often exploit this digital thinking mode by dividing topics into simplistic either-or statements such as, "I am right, vote for me. My opponent is wrong, don't vote for him." Political issues invariably contain elements of uncertainty that cover a whole spectrum of confusing facts and thoughts. This inherent ambiguity and ambivalence requires tremendous thinking effort on the part of the voter. For the politicians, analogue discourse certainly does not fit into brief sound bites. For the electorate, colluding with the politicians by allowing them to frame issues in binary terms makes voting decisions easier. The danger arises that voters can then be digitally divided and conquered.

Contemporary news items dealing with the "war on terror" are rife with examples of digital thinking. If the enemy is the evildoer, it follows that we are the good ones. The foe needs only to be converted or destroyed. Since by definition the position of the others can have no validity, discussions and negotiations are completely unnecessary. "You are either with us or against us." Only the capitulation of the others counts. And so polarization increase. Binary/digital thinking permits no middle ground.

Appropriate analogue thinking, though, carries a heavy price. We forfeit ease of thought, absolute certainty, and righteous comfort and must tolerate uncertainty, discomfort, confusion, and ambivalence. Gone is the solace of clear absolutes; it is replaced by troublesome awareness of the relative and of mixed feelings. The ability to tolerate ambivalence, therefore, defines maturity. *Confusion and uncertainty are midwives to the birth of the Adult.*

With so many adults operating in modes of absolute binary thinking, the world seems populated by large children with very few adults around, as evidenced by the most cursory review of the day's news at the local, national, and international levels. For all its sophistication, the world too often seems like a sandbox filled with squabbling kids. But in the sandbox of today's world, squabbling frequently proves fatal. Our contemporary anxiety is that only the sand, turned to radioactive glass, will remain.

Autonomy versus Immature Dependence

Helpless at birth, the infant depends totally on his mother or other caretaker for survival. This natural condition, referred to as *immature dependence*, becomes incorporated within the child as the first real model for relationships with others. With "good enough" parenting, the child gradually matures, developing a healthy sense of self that allows him to grow to adulthood. He is capable of establishing satisfying relationships which are characterized as mutually respectful and growth-enhancing. He does not fear that a relationship will diminish him in any way. As an *autonomous* adult, he can take care of himself *and* be *maturely dependent* in intimate relationships.

On the other hand, if a person's early experiences were traumatic, painful, or demeaning, he will harbor fears that future close relationships will bring more of the same, and, at the same time, he will be drawn to those who perpetuate the familiar. Therefore, as a defense against having to experience the helpless state of immature dependence once again, he may opt to maintain an *independent* posture. Independence—the ability to stand on one's own two feet—may be an admirable characteristic, but not in close relationships when it prevents intimacy. A person who asserts his independence in a close relationship avoids intimacy; he becomes a *pseudo-adult*, appearing competent and capable but remaining emotionally immature and guarded. Conversely, if he wishes to have greater intimacy, he may pay the price of engaging either in a relationship in which he feels diminished—as he did in childhood—or one in which he himself denigrates his partner. In either case, he is immaturely dependent on his partner.

In an immature dependent relationship one party is dominant (parent) and the other is subservient (child). In healthy interactions, the goal is to reach mutuality—both partners are respected and seen as worthwhile. But for adults who reestablish immature childhood connections, dominance and subservience are simply two sides of the same dysfunctional coin. The dominant-parent partner, identifying with some controlling and perhaps even punitive significant other from childhood, imposes helpless, immature dependence onto the subservient-child partner in an attempt to escape his own fears of helplessness. This process is called *identification with the aggressor.*

A common illustration of this phenomenon in childhood is seen after a child has been to the doctor for a shot. Playing doctor on returning home, he jabs a pencil into a younger sibling's arm. In this way, the child tries to control the helpless feelings he experienced at the doctor's office. The Kapos in the Nazi concentration camps provide a more extreme and horrific example of adults acting similarly. They were prisoners appointed by Hitler's Schutzstaffel (S.S.) corps to police the other inmates. The Kapos, identifying with the aggressors, often acted more cruelly than their guards to please the Nazis and avoid either feeling helpless or themselves becoming victims. There is a myriad of ways this dynamic plays out in ordinary relationships.

Immature dependence may result from overindulgence as well as neglect and abuse. A person who was indulged and discouraged from growing up as a child may, as an adult, seek out an immature dependent relationship by finding someone willing to be the long-suffering, all-giving caretaker. This partner continues to enable the person to avoid assuming appropriate adult responsibilities. Immature dependence, whatever its variation, goes hand in hand with binary thinking. The couple sees the dominant partner as all good or strong and the subservient partner as bad or weak, which results in a common form of human interaction: the *power play*. Relationships operating in such a way are defined as having a winner/loser, master/slave, or strong/weak dyad. People describing their relationships frequently use these ordinary terms, emphasizing just how common power play is.

In stark contrast to the power play is the much rarer mode of human interaction: the *love play*. This does not refer to the erotic but to people engaging one another with mutual respect, consideration, care, and understanding. Fairbairn eloquently said that our goal in significant relationships is to grow from the state of natural immature dependence to that of mature dependence.[5]

Individuals who are capable of truly loving behavior function in an *autonomous* state. Autonomy, the ability to stand on one's own *and* be intimate, contrasts with psychological *independence*, which is a defense against returning to the initial primordial state of immature dependence. The independent person perceives himself as being able *either* to stand on his own *or* feel diminished by closeness. He may look like a functioning adult, but he operates in the Child state because of his crucial need for emotional distance. Such individuals may be referred to as *pseudo-adults*.

Growing from the Child state of immature dependence to the Adult state of autonomy with the ability to form maturely dependent relationships represents the central task all of us have in life. The following schematic illustrates this idea.

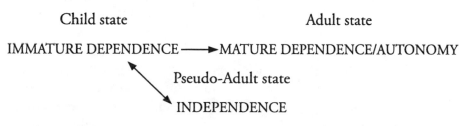

Figure 2-1 From Immature To Mature Dependence

Vulnerability versus Helplessness

To grow, achieve autonomy, and develop mature dependence, we must dare to be vulnerable. In childhood we experienced *vulnerability* as being synonymous with *helplessness*, thereby emotionally welding together these two very different phenomena. When we realize that this perceived equivalency no longer holds true, change becomes possible. Philosophically, it is conceivable that an adult can be profoundly vulnerable and yet never helpless. The difference is straightforward. A child has no options; an **A**dult *always* has. For an adult, choice helps to make the crucial distinction between functioning emotionally as an **A**dult and functioning as a **C**hild.

For example, imagine you choose to fly across the country in a commercial airplane in spite of a known, though improbable, chance of danger. At 35,000 feet, the pilot announces trouble, and the plane is clearly going to crash. Powerful emotions naturally rush forward and precipitate a regressive pull to the past. You feel trapped and helpless—the experience of the **C**hild. But you are also potentially aware that as an adult you had made a reasonable choice in taking the flight. With that choice you recognized the possibility of some inherent risk, though there was little probability that an accident would occur since flying remains the safest form of travel. Death may now be imminent and inevitable. The only question is how you will choose to die. Will it be as an **A**dult or as a **C**hild?

I do not mean to seem naive or ridiculous in using such an extreme illustration. Consider the importance of this philosophical postulate: It is the singular sense of choice that allows us to be vulnerable yet never trapped, hopeless, or helpless, even when circumstances occur that may reignite such feelings from childhood. There is a world of difference between what we may feel and what the facts are, just as there is a world of difference between childhood and adulthood. Farfetched as the foregoing example may seem, I would credit those who fought back against the terrorists on United Flight 93 on September 11, 2001 with making such a distinction.

How many people, as children, lost a pet they loved? It hurt terribly. The child could feel only utter helplessness in the face of such loss. Those past feelings may remain with the child as he grows up and influence him not to want another pet. Never getting another pet guarantees that he will never feel the same devastation from losing it, but the pleasure of having one would be sacrificed. Losing a significant person such as a parent or sibling magnifies the child's devastation. As an adult he may have considerable problems with relationships as he tries to find some optimum ratio between intimacy, for the desired pleasures, and safety, for the avoidance of potential loss.

Choice, Competency, Resources

The Child distinguishes no difference between vulnerability and helplessness, because to him these emotions feel the same. Our ability as Adults to acknowledge the vast distinction between these two perceptions makes it possible for us to change and function primarily in the Adult state. In the process, we must take meaningful chances, face reasonable risks, and know that we will no longer be emotionally destroyed or devastated by the experiences. Not daring to pursue what we Want chains us to the past and prevents us from reaching our potentials. Without accepting the possibility of loss, we cannot love. To love, we must be willing to give a hostage to fortune (fate).[6] Otherwise the Child's fears will hold the adult's present pleasures captive. Knowing that we have choices and that being vulnerable is no longer the same as being helpless, we can cast off the old chains and free ourselves to pursue what we Want.

Rachel Naomi Ramen proposed that we have the power to *choose the inevitable*, a crucial concept.[7] Ramen described a woman who was rushed by her doctor and family into having surgery to remove a malignancy. After the surgery, she became depressed and sought therapy. Her perception of having no choice generated the feeling of being a helpless, trapped child, which contributed to the depression. She felt that she had not made the choice of having surgery herself; rather everyone else had made it for her, just as caring parents do for a helpless child. She realized that she was not helpless, nor was she so foolish as to think of not having surgery. Does this mean that she had no choice? Not at all. Her therapy allowed her to recognize that she could choose the inevitable. By doing so, she appreciated herself as being an Adult and not a hopeless, helpless Child. The difference is in knowing that choice exists.

Earlier I described a study showing that the agony of rejection from a group to which a person believes he must belong registers in the same brain regions as does physical pain. Aleksandr Solzhenitsyn described feeling free for the first time in his adult life when he was locked up in the gulag.[8] He recognized that other prisoners desperately felt that they had to be part of the Soviet system, represented by the guards. They perceived no other options. Therefore, as though they were children with parents, the prisoners gave the guards power they did not otherwise have. Solzhenitsyn realized that he had a choice: Allow the government to think for him, or continue to think for himself. He could and did choose to dissociate himself from the Soviet system. That ended the guards' emotional leverage. He was in the gulag but felt he was free.

Freud said that the goal of psychotherapy is "where id is, ego shall be."[9] I would like to paraphrase that statement by saying the goal of therapy is *where no choice was, choice shall be.* The implementation of that knowledge changes the Child to the Adult.

I do not endorse the concept that we create our own world and are responsible for everything that happens in it. Certainly there are external occurrences not under our control, but what *is* exclusively in our domain is *choosing* how we will experience those occurrences. John Milton, in *Paradise Lost,* observed: "The mind is its own place, and to itself can make a heav'n of hell or a hell of heav'n."[10] The first century CE Roman philosopher Epictetus said, "It is not events which disturb me, rather it is my perception of those events."[11] Not just an abstract notion, this is a philosophical truth worth remembering. We may not control the events themselves, but we always control how we choose to perceive the events. Our choices distinguish each of us—if ultimately only to ourselves—as being in the Adult and not in the Child state.

As an individual values his accumulating experiences, he develops greater awareness of his competence. While his achievements grow, so does his recognition of internal and external resources. Ideally, one raises a child by giving him age- and ability-appropriate tasks to solve through trial and error, providing encouragement, and assuring him that he is not a failure even if he fails to solve the problems. He will learn which attempted solutions work and why those that failed did not. With no sense of failure, he will not fear trying again.

When the parent states, "I can't predict what will come your way in life, but I'm confident that whatever it is, you'll do your best, learn from it, and grow as a result of the experience," the child develops the confidence needed to deal with the inevitable problems that arise throughout life. Lincoln reputedly said that a man might fail many times but is a failure only if he gives up trying. Perhaps apocryphal is the story of Thomas Edison being asked if he was discouraged that it took numerous laborious experiments to reach the significant one. "Oh, no," he said, "I learned 10,000 ways that didn't work."

Alone versus Lonely

In the Adult state, we acknowledge our inner strengths, resources, and choices. People who experience themselves as Adults never feel emotionally lonely. They may be alone, but they are not lonely, because they are with themselves and appreciate the good company. They may strongly desire companionship, but they do not feel diminished without it. In contrast, a person who lacks a sense of inner value evokes the Child, which carries with it the associated emotions of loneliness and the fear of being "home alone." That person fails to appreciate that even though no one else may be present, *he* is—and he cannot feel whole without others. How often might a caller ask a child answering the telephone, "Is anyone there?"

"No," comes the reply.

Empathy versus Sympathy

I do not employ *empathy* and *sympathy* in the traditional, dictionary sense. I define empathy as the concern a person has about another person's plight when he, the observer, feels whole and healthy himself—the Adult. Sympathy, on the other hand, I define as a person's concern about another person's problem when he, the observer, lacks self-value and depends on that other person to provide him with a sense of wholeness—the Child.

For example, an adult child of troubled parents—feeling hurt by, dependant on, and disappointed in the parents—sees cutting off the relationship as his only option. Instead, he could learn to appreciate himself as a person separate from his parents and maintain contact as an empathic observer—a survivor, not a victim. Even as we may have no sympathy for a criminal, we can have great empathy for the circumstances that led that person to choose to commit crimes.

Perhaps a metaphor will further help to distinguish the way I am using these terms. Empathy is what you feel for the captain of a ship that is sinking when you perceive yourself being securely aboard your own vessel—the Adult state. Sympathy is what you feel for the captain of a ship that is sinking when you perceive yourself as being a passenger on the sinking vessel—the Child state. Even if the airplane about to crash or the ship about to sink were real and not just metaphorical circumstances, a person can still choose to function in the Adult state (empathic and vulnerable) and not in the Child state (sympathetic and helpless).

Desire versus Desperation

People frequently evaluate behavior as mature or immature. Who has not had the experience of labeling someone as behaving "like a child" or himself being so labeled? However, the external behavior alone does not necessarily reveal whether it is the **Adult** or **Child** in action. Rather, the motivation behind the behavior determines the state. *Desire motivates the Adult; desperation drives the Child.* This is a crucial distinction. Certainly both feelings can coexist, in which case it is important to recognize which state predominates.

Take, for example, a couple engaging in a sexual relationship. There may be desire on one or both partners' parts, but if the woman participates primarily out of fear that she will not otherwise be liked or accepted, or the man out of concern that he must avoid being seen as inadequate, it is desperation that motivates their behavior. Performing an act of kindness to avoid being seen as bad differs from performing the same act because one wants to. The act remains the same, as does the importance to the recipient. Desperation, predicated on self-negation or the perception of not being okay, distinguishes the first act from the second, which is motivated by desire.

Action based on desperation never changes the **Child**'s underlying sense of self. The action serves only to delay any dreaded judgment until another day. "I know I have three strikes against me before I even get to bat. If I hit a home run and the crowd cheers, it was just a fluke, and I fooled everyone—until I come to bat again." Whatever the external success may be, actions motivated by desperation count solely as temporarily evading the "fraud squad." Only in the **Adult** state ("I know I am okay") can gratification from a positive action be meaningfully incorporated. Think of how often we have difficulty simply saying "thank you" to a compliment, because it evokes some residual **Child** feeling of unworthiness.

Envy versus Jealousy

In the **Child** state, we often have great difficulty acknowledging the successes of others, as though such achievements serve only to expose our own inadequacies. We react by experiencing *jealousy* and perhaps even expressing antipathy toward the successful person. Jealousy means that we feel diminished by other people's accomplishments, and therefore we in turn must negate or diminish those achievements.

In the **Adult** state, we may feel *envy* of another person's successes, but we recognize that we could, with application, achieve the same or better. If not, we have our own unique strengths and abilities that are of value even if very different from those of the envied others. From this perspective, envy does not necessitate loathing of self or the other.

Want versus Need

I use the common words Want and Need specifically to describe two different characteristics of the **Adult** and **Child**, and indicate their special connotation by capitalizing them. The concept of Want is used to express the **Adult's** desires for a life free from past conflicts. In contrast, Need expresses the entire constellation of cues associated with survival that we learn in childhood. The **Child** desperately holds onto these familiar cues that provide the feeling of home. If the **Child's** Needs are also desired by the **Adult**, they transform into Wants. If they are not desired and are still imbued with life-sustaining meaning, they become problems that cannot be ignored. These problems reside in the **Child** part of the self and become activated when the adult is threatened with change. Then *the battle lines of emotional conflict are drawn between the Child's Needs and the Adult's Want.*

The psychologically derived Needs of the **Child**, however, differ from the fundamental, biological processes associated with physical survival. Survival imperatives that evolved from the reptilian brain drive the behavior of all living organisms. They are most evident when safety and security are threatened, as, for example, when natural or human-generated disasters occur. In a shipwreck, convention dictates that women and children be rescued first, but how often do the men jump in ahead of the others? How often did gas station attendants during a fuel shortage have to wear sidearms for protection from the fuel-hungry? Such circumstances give credence to the observation that a thin veneer of civility covers our animal origins. Respectfully, I believe it was this fundamental drive that allowed many in the Nazi concentration camps to survive their ordeal, but it is not these biological imperatives that I am addressing when using the term Need.

Inherently, Needs are a child's emotional survival mechanisms. In that sense they are positive, because without them the child would perish. Needs are always framed in binary/digital terms—all or none—because they come from early childhood experiences. Many of the child's Needs may also be desired when he is a grown-up, in which case they become transformed into the Wants of the **A**dult state. For example, a child who grows up in a family that values honesty, integrity, and fairness incorporates those cues as aspects of what defines home and what characterizes him as a member of his family. Conflicts arise and emotional work becomes necessary when what the **C**hild Needs *differs* from what the **A**dult Wants.

When confronted with circumstances that are horrible, we experience great discomfort and make every possible effort to reestablish familiar, desired conditions. Referring to the barbarous situation of the Nazi concentration camps, Viktor Frankl said, "The best of us did not survive."[12] He meant that those who could not tolerate the degradation died. Holding values about life that they would not compromise, they preferred death to the camp's horrendous reality. We can readily identify with those prisoners' imperative to reestablish common decency and human dignity or else die, literally or figuratively. Their Wants were of greater significance under these circumstances than was survival itself.

A patient of mine who survived the concentration camps described his grief over the death of his own decency. Every night for sixty years the image of what he did to stay alive haunted him. He stole a day's ration of food, consisting of a small piece of stale bread, from another prisoner. The other prisoner died the next day. The patient felt he had forfeited his human values for animal survival and had great difficulty coming to peace with his action. His biological imperative to survive superseded the decency he Wanted.

We admire people who try to behave with dignity in the face of barbarous conditions, but we find it difficult to comprehend the reverse situation: People who desperately try to reestablish brutal conditions under decent circumstances. But we must do so if we are to understand the dynamics of emotional conflicts that result from the mobilization of powerful Need forces. Take as an example the abused child, placed in his wished-for caring foster home, who acts out, sorely tempting the new parents to punish him. The **C**hild state's emotional intensity and the Need to maintain familiar cues, even when those cues are destructive, explain his provocative behavior. In states of emotional conflict, the intensity of Need may overwhelm what the adult desires.

The Path of Growth

The following graph summarizes healthy growth from childhood through adolescence to adulthood. It illustrates an emerging **A**dult—

symbolized by the smaller font size—who resides in every child, though the Child state predominates in childhood. In adolescence, the transitional state both psychologically and physiologically between childhood and adulthood, a greater Adult emerges in addition to the Child component. Both are present and competing which contributes to the natural adolescent turmoil.

Just as there is an aspect of the Adult in every child, there exists in every adult a latent residual Child, along with a potentially active, realized Adult. In the healthy adult, the Adult state predominates—but always with an element of the residual Child, containing any unresolved conflicts from the past.

Childhood   Adolescence   Adulthood

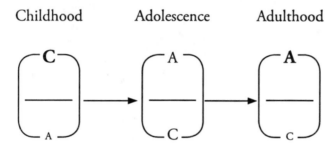

Figure 2-2 Healthy Growth

In childhood, we incorporate vital Need cues that signal our feelings of connectedness and safety. As we grow, Needs that are no longer necessary may evolve and potentially become expressed as desired Wants. Conflict arises when we tenaciously pursue past Needs that are no longer vital and are antithetical to what we Want in the present. It is in the colliding interface between what the Adult Wants and the Child Needs that human psychological turmoil arises. To let go of such Needs, *to break the chains that keep us from what we Want,* is to risk going through a profound void—the zero—before we can have what we Want. Exploring and explaining why this can be such a titanic struggle for some people and how that conflict manifests itself is the topic of the following chapters.

CHAPTER THREE

The Child/Adult States in Action

In its earliest days, psychoanalytic theorizing focused on the idea that we are born with sexual and aggressive drives and that our primary goal is to discharge these drives. Significant others were viewed as secondary, serving to guide the discharge in a socially appropriate fashion. Supplanting this notion was the overarching awareness that the newborn must make a connection with a caretaker. Significant others thus became of primary importance. The nature of the bond formed is secondary and we will take whatever we can get in order to survive.

The Uniqueness of Learning as a Child

The child learns what constitutes the necessary connections with significant others that assure his survival and, especially, how to maintain those bonds. This knowledge forms the Need cues, which are learned under unique conditions that are theoretically confined to childhood: *optionlessness* and *idealization*. The infant has no viable alternative for the circumstances into which he is born. He cannot say, "I have assessed the situation, recognize I picked troubled parents, and am packing my pabulum and moving next door, where the folks seem much nicer." Therefore he has to accept whatever his family provides. When we have no options, we tend to idealize our situation and convince ourselves that what we have is the best possible. This is an emotional rather than intellectual reckoning based on the child's reality which makes such initial learning extremely difficult to extinguish.

Our internal struggles and emotional conflicts arise from this *idealized optionlessness* and become tenaciously perpetuated. Not only does the child learn how to connect under this unique paradigm, but he also learns who he is and how to function in the world. The child's Needs become imbued with the intense emotional, life-or-death necessity to perpetuate the familiar. That makes change not only difficult but frightening. A person mindful of both the desire to grow and the threat that growth represents might think, "I don't mind change—as long as nothing is different!"

Berne spoke with brilliant clarity when he said that being a child is like being a midget in the land of giants. We have to believe that the giants know where they are stepping. If we are stepped on, we have to believe that it was because we were underfoot and not because they don't know what they are doing. Otherwise we cannot rest.[1] This can be illustrated by a young child's spontaneous assumption of blame for Mommy and Daddy's divorce because, he claims, "I didn't eat my vegetables," or "I wet the bed." The child attempts to take on the parents' problems. If he—not the parents—is the bad one, he creates the illusion of having ideal parents. This is not altruism in action. With perfect parents, there will be perfect safety for the child. The illusion seems worth the cost.

As we grow up, we either gradually resolve and relinquish our childhood Needs, transforming them into our **A**dult Wants, or we retain them as unresolved conflicts, and they form our **C**hild state. When what we as adults desire conflicts with our **C**hild Needs, an inner tension develops. Resolving the conflict requires emotional work, for without resolution, the survival-imbued emotional cues (Needs), the maintaining of the old and familiar, weigh more heavily and tip the scales to the past. The adult's present aspirations are sacrificed.

The "weight" of Need intensity varies with the individual with the specifics of the circumstances, as well as over time. Very significant factors, such as having a tenuous sense of self (ego strength), choosing a mate, or any other significant event (birth of a child, loss of employment, death of a parent, etc.) tilt the person all the more toward maintaining the past. Over time, with accumulating growth-enhancing experiences, the adult gains greater maturity, which strengthens his **A**dult ability to counterbalance these old forces.

Maintaining Predictability

Our urgent wish to be able to predict what will happen in the future prompts us to hold onto what was familiar in the past. The popularity of astrology, fortunetelling, and palm reading, or some variation of these, can be seen in virtually every culture in recorded history. Most people would like to know what is going to happen in the future as a way of making present decisions easier. More profoundly, our awareness that we will eventually die creates a paradoxical urgency to be reassured that the familiar will continue—the Child's Needs—lest we die. A person may try to predict the future by rigidly keeping the present the same as the past in the hope that tomorrow will be like today, modeled on yesterday. Obviously, if we follow this formula, we have very little flexibility when facing new circumstances. A person controlled by his Child masquerades as an adult.

In humankind's thousands of years of recorded history, war has been reported for all but a few hundred years. Civil War General W. T. Sherman's expression "war is hell" seems incomplete. "War is hell, but who knows what the alternative would be like?" appears more accurate. That is, society resorts to the familiar, even if painful and destructive, rather than risking a new, healthier solution to conflicts. The classic British film *King of Hearts* depicts inmates of an asylum taking over a city that has been abandoned in anticipation of a battle during World War I. After watching the English and German soldiers annihilate one another, the inmates quietly slip back into the asylum, wondering who the truly insane ones are.

Only since the development of atomic weapons has a limbo state come about, because mutually assured destruction is too horrific to contemplate. This temporary lull on the world's stage has ended. We have returned to the tried-and-true weapons and even attempted to develop battlefield nuclear devices. Those who try to force their perceived truths onto others who believe differently by using such weapons add to the nightmare.

I make these societal references to emphasize that what we observe in individuals is also found in the relationships between individuals, among groups of people known as nations, and between states. Isaiah's prophecy (Isaiah 2:4) remains woefully unfulfilled: "They shall beat their swords into plowshares, their spears into pruning knives; nation shall not lift up sword against nation nor ever again learn war." That will be the time the Adult prevails over the Child.

On Prejudice

The ubiquity of prejudice reveals the residual childhood conflicts of people manifested in society. When as children we remove the aspects of our parents that we perceive to be bad and internalize the badness within ourselves, we create the myth of having all-good parents. The bad now resides in us. Consider this metaphor: The parents feed their child a little poison with his food. The child can choose to starve or to eat, denying there is anything amiss, and thus ingest the poison. He relieves his anxiety about having parents who serve him poison by seeing them as good and focusing on how to live as the one who is sick (bad). He can deny that he is damaged, fantasizing instead that he can dump the poison onto others, who will now be the contaminated ones. As long as he keeps his distance from those he has tainted, he can maintain the hoax of self-purity. Thus prejudice is born.

An eighteenth-century English explorer came upon a paradisiacal island in the Pacific. He fired his cannon at the beach before he and his party landed, considerably impressing the natives. He described the people he met as being very childlike and "totally free of prejudice." They fancied his cannon and traded goods and provisions to obtain one along with ammunition and instructions on its use. Subsequent voyagers found that the explorer had met only the lowlanders. Another group lived inland, high on a mountain. The lowlanders and the mountain people were clearly descendents of the original founders of the island, yet the two groups were constantly at war. It is easy to see how handy a cannon was for these "totally free of prejudice" people in their battle with those who held the high ground.[2]

Gentlemen's Agreement is a 1947 movie about a journalist who pretends to be Jewish in order to research anti-Semitism. He was interested in knowing what the experience would be like of suddenly being excluded from places and relationships simply by "revealing" his religious affiliation. Sometime after seeing this film for the first time, I wrote these words:

How convenient others are by differing in some way.
Makes it so much easier my inner problems to display.
When I am upset, and things don't seem to be working out,
Someone's handy, you can bet, against whom I can spout.
There are religions of every creed, skin colors, mores by the lot.

> Paying the Golden Rule no heed, I just pick a group in which I'm not.
> By hating very willfully, this whole group I can mar.
> Solves my problems skillfully. How convenient others are.

To eliminate prejudice, we must recognize the good in others, which also helps diminish our anxiety about strangers.[3] But this requires our willingness to take back the sense of badness we originally tried to get rid of by dumping it onto them. There are many horrendous examples of how difficult this can be. When the economy of Indonesia sank in 1965, so did the decency of many Indonesians, who turned their rage onto the ethnic Chinese in their communities. The same tale is told by the terrible reality of the Nazi Holocaust and the conflicts between Tutsis and Hutus, Irish Catholics and Protestants, Israelis and Arabs, Christians and Muslims, and Hindus and Sikhs. And the list goes on. We try to dispose of our own pain by inflicting it on others. All too readily we replace insecurities and self-doubt with the certainty that it is the others who are defective. Denying self-contempt, we can feel superior by heaping the disdain on "them." Tolerance has never come naturally.[4] The word *tolerance* is derived from the Latin *tolerantia*, which means *the capacity to endure pain or adversity.* That is what is necessary to reclaim the painful aspects of ourselves that we project onto others.

If prejudice actually worked in eliminating our self-loathing it would perhaps have something to commend it. But it does not even accomplish that. The awareness that the sense of badness originated within us may be gone, but not the internal, self-negating feelings that still act against us, even as we project those feelings onto others. The terms of Germany's surrender after World War I, which left that nation humiliated and demoralized, demonstrates this. Rallying around the notion of being the Master Race still left an internal, collective, unacknowledged psyche of inferiority, requiring the displacement of such painful feelings onto others: Homosexuals, Romas, Jews, and the physically and mentally handicapped. Owning one's pain and not displacing it on another is by its very definition painful and vigorously defended against. Therefore people often have great difficulties in abandoning their prejudices.

Imagine a man watching from a distance as two boys who are excitedly arguing in a sand lot begin to tussle with each other. Suddenly one of them pulls away and runs to get a shovel. Returning, he vigorously digs a hole. Dropping the shovel, he re-engages in the tussle and succeeds in pushing the other boy into the hole and holding him there. Baffled, the man finally goes over and asks what the argument could possibly be about to account for such strange behavior. "We were arguing about who is taller," said the boy holding the other down, "and I just won." Whereupon the man shakes his head and asks, "Wouldn't it have been easier just to get a chair and stand on it?" Great energy is often expended in trying to diminish others rather than enhance oneself.

The Stockholm Syndrome

Theoretically, the earliest paradigm for a child's learning—that of idealized optionlessness—should never extend beyond childhood. In reality, it often does. In a hostage situation, the captor controls whether the captive lives or dies. The incredible stress this creates for some can precipitate a regression to the past. Being a hostage replicates being a child, with the captor as the parent who has the power to decide whether the child will live or die. A susceptible person, feeling helpless and perceiving no options, may idealize the symbolic parent, the all-good person, now viewed as unappreciated by others.

In a Swedish bank, hostages were held for a prolonged time before being liberated by the authorities. Surprisingly, some who were freed began to offer justifications for their captors' behavior, vociferously expressing displeasure with the authority's actions. This surprising outcome has been observed in other hostage situations as well. It was part of the explanation offered in defense of Patty Hurst's actions of idealizing and subsequently joining her Symbionese Liberation Army abductors. A capricious kidnapper pointing an Uzi submachine gun at a hostage is a potent, even if unconscious, symbol of the life-and-death power a parent has over a child.

This phenomenon of idealizing the captor is so striking and seen so often that it has been given a name: the Stockholm syndrome.[5] Cult leaders induce a similar regression by cultivating a parent-child dependency in their members, often depriving them of sleep and protein. This produces a pliable, compliant, Child-like state. No beatings, torture, or threats are required.

Of course, not everyone is prone to such regression. Those with a strong sense of themselves as Adults are much less likely to succumb. However, with significant stress, we are all capable of falling back into our Child state. That we regress is less important than how long the regression lasts and how debilitating it is. As we develop greater mastery over ourselves, our regressions—if they take place at all—tend to be of short duration and diminished intensity.

As an intern, I vividly recall making surgical rounds and visiting a sixty-five-year-old woman who had just had abdominal surgery. She had left Estonia at age five and had not spoken her native language or heard it spoken for sixty years. As we removed the dressings to examine the incision, we discovered that the wound had dehisced; it had split wide open. The patient had a ringside seat to her own gaping abdominal cavity. Suddenly she expressed her horror—in Estonian! Her capacity to speak that language stunned her as much as it amazed us after she explained how long it had been since she had uttered any words in Estonian. This was certainly an indelible marker for the power of regression when a person is under stress.

The Power of Choice

As noted earlier, if the pull of the past becomes greater than our strength in the present, we regress to an earlier state. In other words, when the Child state rules the adult, we operate as if we were living in the past and not in the present. The fact that an adult's present can become emotionally displaced by his past gives testimony to the primordial power of childhood Needs and with those Needs the accompanying sense of helplessness.

I cannot overemphasize the importance of appreciating that we always have choices, even if what we choose is the inevitable. The awareness of choice is the antidote to the corrosive perception of helplessness. *Choice obviates Child.*

A young woman was taken captive by four men and driven to a remote hillside housing development. The men dragged her onto the raw wood floor of a house under construction and took turns raping her. She was able to say to herself, "It is inevitable that my body will be abused, but I am more than just my body. I must do nothing that will prompt them to push me into the canyon below when they have finished. I will survive. And I must memorize every aspect of their appearance and their car to be able to make a police report." Amazingly, her feigned helplessness lulled the perpetrators into not seeing her as a threat. They left her on the floor and drove away. She was able to give accurate enough details to result in arrests and subsequent convictions. Though stark, this example of a remarkable young woman powerfully illustrates our ability to counter regression and exercise choice. The woman, while extremely vulnerable and experiencing feelings of helplessness, knew that she was not helpless. She had choices, including the inevitable, which empowered her.

People who operate with fundamentalist ideas of absolutism function in their **Child** state. They presume there are no other choices than the "correct" ones they have made; all others are wrong. Though they look grown-up, they behave like large children masquerading as adults. These pseudo-adults function with digital/binary thinking alone. In this sense, the radically left-wing Weathermen and the radically right-wing John Birch Society resemble each other more than either group would care to acknowledge. Both insist that their views are the only correct ones. All absolutists—whether religious, political, or philosophical—act similarly by shunning uncertainty and ambivalence and clinging to the givens from the past. People acting in their **Adult** state, on the other hand, examine their beliefs, recognize options, and make choices that do not necessitate absolutes.

Advocates of the religious idea called *intelligent design*, with their complete disdain for Darwin's scientific theory of evolution, illustrate their Need for having a fixed certainty, unquestioned answers, and no other options about creation than their own unique biblical interpretations. This is especially egregious because they espouse their religious beliefs in pseudoscientific terms that entirely lack any valid scientific basis while denying the overwhelming evidence verifying Darwinism.[6] For them, faith must trump fact in order to maintain the security of their beliefs. Uncertainty is too threatening.

Galileo's affirmation of Copernicus's discovery that the Sun, not the Earth, is the center of our planetary system had to be quelled because the ramifications became much too frightening. Restive populations could disrupt ruling powers. Entire prior conceptualizations would be undermined. The agony of uncertainty would reign. In the natural development of a child's thinking, the early characteristic of hungering for absolutes transcends historic time, making it seem that, for some, nothing has changed since Galileo—or anytime earlier. Fixed certainties serve as anesthetics, dispelling the pain but dulling the senses.

I mention these cultural examples in preparation for the next chapter's discussion of the book's central theme: Breaking free, which entails the risk of letting go of past limiting beliefs to find new awareness in the present. Acceptance of uncertainty, and the willingness to test hypotheses, characterizes the **A**dult state. No one said it would be easy. The chains from childhood securely hold us in a predictable, familiar world.

On the marquee of a neighborhood church, the minister posted his sermon for the following Sunday: "What If I Should Awake Before I Die?" In that title, the pastor captured the ease with which so many people remain asleep in the familiar, predictable sameness of the past and never awaken to the present—to say nothing of the future.

We are awake and in the **A**dult state when we freely recognize that choices exist. Doing so, however, immediately threatens the status quo and evokes **C**hild Needs and resistance to change. This is true even when we know intellectually that what we Want is better than those Needs to which we so fervently cling emotionally. The anthem of the insecure is, "Don't confuse me with the facts, my mind is made up."

Wanting and Having

Wanting something is an entirely different experience than actually *having* what is wanted—another paradox. Take, for example, the person who wants to be wealthy. He may labor assiduously to reach that goal. When he reaches it, a curious struggle occurs. He knows how to *try* to be wealthy, but he has no idea how to *be* wealthy. I realize that in response to this statement many might say, "Just try me." Yet those who have become wealthy frequently do not know how to enjoy their wealth. Lottery winners rarely feel more content with their lives after winning; some even squander their new-found wealth so that they may quickly return to their old, but familiar, lives. The history of families with great wealth dissipated by the third generation also speaks to this phenomenon.

As another example, picture a young girl arriving home from school to a father who greets her unshaven, in his underwear, drunk, and throwing beer bottles at her as she walks in the door. Every night she goes to bed beseeching whatever powers that be to intercede and fix Daddy. One night her pleadings are somehow answered. She arrives home the next day to find a sober, dressed, shaved, welcoming, loving father. What does she do? Well, first she goes outside to check the address. Is this the right house? Then something very curious occurs. She begins to attempt to provoke her father, to upset him enough that he will resume the very behaviors she abhors. She has what she Wants but has lost what she Needs—the familiar, or that which told her she was home. Every therapist has seen the resistant emergence of significant others when a patient actually makes the desired changes. No matter how much they want the patient to change, predictability must not be sacrificed. The power of the young girl's Need for the familiar overwhelmed her desire for the new. She must set things "right" so she can return to wishing for change. As do so many other children in similar situations—commonly but not exclusively female— she may grow to adulthood thrilled finally to be free of her father, only to find herself drawn back into an abusive relationship, this time with a husband.

A sailor rescued a man who had been adrift for many days after his ship had sunk in high seas. The man had survived by clinging desperately to a piece of driftwood, the shattered remains of a large wooden barrel. As the survivor was taken aboard the rescue vessel, the sailor could not pry loose the man's hold on the wood even though he was safe. Naturally, being saved was absolutely what he wanted, but emotionally it meant giving up the now worthless piece of driftwood that he had imbued with all the emotions associated with his survival. He clung tenaciously to the idealized stave and feared the consequence of losing it. Certainly this is not the experience of everyone rescued at sea, but it illustrates how difficult it is, even to the point of seeming absurd and irrational, to let go of what once represented survival.

Some people tolerate inordinately difficult circumstances even when to outward appearances it would be so easy for them to improve their lot by acting differently. Those people learned as children to pay a dollar for every nickel they got—and be glad for the nickel. That paradigm becomes incorporated as a cue for connectedness, an aspect of their Need system, and trumps clear expressions of Wants. This does not occur because they do not desire to be okay. Everyone does. It is nonsense to say that some people do not want to be well. It simply means that they learned in childhood to tolerate—even Need—such adverse circumstances to feel at home.

Change

Therapy, or growth by any other name or means, helps us to function in the present, unencumbered by the limitations of past perceptions that are no longer desired. Patients may ask their therapists, "Will therapy help me change?" It is a trick question, because the part the patient usually wishes to change through therapy is not *he* himself but *his past*. If the painful past were just a bad dream from which the person could be awakened, the pain would go away. The notion of "healing the inner child," though poetically beautiful, is no more possible than giving someone a new past. That cannot be done, but it often constitutes the longing that is hidden in the agenda of a relationship, be it with a mate, a friend, or a therapist.

So how is change possible? Every child deserves to have a healthy, supportive, nurturing childhood. Too bad that this just does not happen often enough. Only by mourning what could have been, what one deserved to have had as a child but did not get, can the **A**dult emerge. Often we try to be whole by ignoring the hole in us, that part that feels painful and unfulfilled. Not surprising, then, that we are left fragmented. Marcel Proust eloquently said, "We are healed of a suffering only by experiencing it to the full."[7] Rachel Naomi Ramen concurred: "There is no healing without grieving."[8]

Does this mean that only one road leads to Rome? Absolutely not. The many different therapies available speak to the wide variety of approaches. What they all have in common is the goal of reaching the "Rome" of being an **A**dult. The schematic shown earlier in this chapter can be expanded to illustrate two major paths by which therapies can be categorized. These paths may exist simultaneously to reach the desired goal; one does not exclude the other.

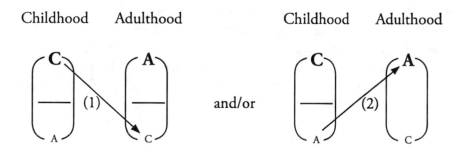

Figure 3-1 Paths of Change

The first path (1), generally that of talk therapy, diminishes the power of the past in the present by recognizing the patient's Need system and how he has clung to and perpetuated it. The **A**dult can then choose which aspects to maintain and incorporate into his Wants and which to discard. Able to empathically understand his **C**hild self, he can now do what was not done for that child—accept and understand him, but with the knowledge that the child's time has passed and can never be other than it was. The Child will always remain a part of the self, but the therapeutic goal is to limit its influence on the patient's present behavior.

Freud understood the value of talking about conflicts. He perceived that his patients' physical symptoms resulted from emotional distress arising in the brain's subcortical regions. The "energy" created by the distress was discharged through the spinal cord to the rest of the body, forming physical symptoms such as paralysis of limbs, fainting spells, and abdominal discomforts—common symptoms in Freud's day. Talking requires engaging the brain's cortex. Freud hypothesized that when the patient verbalizes his problems, energy is shunted to the cortex and therefore is no longer discharged through the body.[9] His observation intuitively anticipated what is now understood about the function of the brain's subcortical limbic lobe—subsequently called the Papez Circuit—in the experience and expression of emotion.

Formulating our thoughts by putting them into words and discussing our concerns and struggles gives us clarity and a sense of command. It is difficult to find solutions to unstated problems. Talking has value even if at times the speaker may be the only one listening. A humorous anecdote comes to mind.

Psychoanalyst Martin Grotjahn hosted Anna Freud during a visit she made to Los Angeles. After they finished dinner, Grotjahn asked if he could have a few minutes for a consultation about a patient he was having trouble understanding. He spoke about the patient for a while and then paused, expecting her reply. Anna Freud apologized and explained that she had been unable to concentrate on anything he had said because of jet lag and exhaustion. Initially disappointed, Grotjahn quickly realized that it was one of the best consultative experiences he had ever had. Why? Because in having to formulate his thoughts, he discovered that he did understand his patient after all.[10]

The first task God gave Adam in the Garden of Eden was to name the animals (Genesis 2:20). This symbolizes the powerful ability of language to create understanding and order. Once named, the unknown loses much of its power to influence beliefs and behaviors. Similarly, we must discover and name our conflicts, no matter how painful they may be, by developing a comprehensive narrative of our lives in order to achieve resolution. Our understanding of and, if necessary, grieving for what should have been but never was—nor ever can be—brings our painful past back into our awareness and allows us to heal.

James Grotstein described a patient's dream that vividly illustrates this struggle to separate "now" from "then." The man dreamed that he was in London and had awakened from his sleep. Dreaming that he could not fall back asleep, he dressed and went for a walk. The streets were deserted, and fog blanketed the area. As he continued toward the illumination of a glowing street lamp, he saw the image of a small boy lying in the gutter. The child, hollow-cheeked and dressed in rags, shivered from the cold. The man deplored the sight of such a desperately bereft child. As he quickened his pace to come closer, he suddenly stopped, emotionally overwhelmed by the realization that the child he saw was the child he had been. He apprehended the totality of the sight, realizing that he could do no more than completely acknowledge the child's pain and then move on—embracing the awareness of what had been. In doing so, he was able to fully appreciate the present.[11]

Referring back to the diagram above, the desired goal in therapy is for the patient to reach a stage in which he primarily functions in the **Adult** state. The first path of reducing the **Child's** influence through verbalization and understanding has been discussed. The second path (indicated by number 2 in the diagram) used by behavioral therapists superimposes **Adult** behavior over **Child** behavior. If the patient can reach a level of functioning that significantly overrides his conflicts, regardless of their origin—without his necessarily understanding them—then he has arrived at the same destination of being an **Adult** that he would have reached in talk therapy. This is when "just say no" works.

Grotjahn offers another example that illustrates this idea of superimposing healthier behavior over conflicted behavior.[12] One day when he was walking from his office a colleague caught up with him and asked if he could have a moment for a consultation. After Grotjahn agreed, the other therapist described the behavior of a patient. Grotjahn slapped his hand to his forehead and said that he thought the man being discussed was likely psychotic and should be hospitalized. Some time later, the two ran into each other again, and the therapist asked if Grotjahn remembered the patient he had described. He said that he did and wondered what had happened to the poor man, whereupon the therapist acknowledged that he had been talking about himself. When Grotjahn had told him how crazy the behavior was he had promptly stopped it.

Both of these paths—behavior change and verbalizing and understanding conflicts—can be followed simultaneously; neither excludes the other. Our ability to use cognitive strengths is a powerful resource in dealing with our emotional problems. However, our thinking capacity must not become subservient to the Child's Needs and undermine the adult's desire to overcome difficulties. For example, a man sits in a sleazy, run-down bar, rationalizing that he is doing everything possible to meet a desirable woman. His behavior and thoughts only perpetuate—and avoid resolving—painful childhood perceptions of himself as unlovable, even though he believes he is making an effort to change.

I have previously stressed how remarkably well our minds prioritize our Needs and commandeer our behavior into fulfilling those Needs. Yet we can be lulled into believing our efforts to change are in the service of resolving conflicts even when we are actually reinforcing them—just like the fellow in the run-down bar.

A caveat is in order: Our thinking, new brain, the neocortex, has evolved much faster than has our primitive, subcortical, survivalist "old" brain, which contains components we have in common with other animals (the limbic and even earlier, reptilian structures). It is a bit like having the most advanced jet propulsion system harnessed to a donkey cart. Every new advance that aids us in constructively reaching greater levels of health and prosperity manifest this remarkable neocortical development. At the same time, these phenomenal cognitive abilities readily become conscripted destructively by the reptilian brain, leading to warfare's remarkable technological advances. The recipient of a blow from the club wielded by another cave dweller is just as dead as the occupant of a high-rise building struck by a ballistic missile. With the simple push of a button, cognitive abilities in the service of primitive purposes have saved us the energy of stalking and clubbing fellow humans, and we get to knock off many more people than we could with club, spear, arrow, or bullet. Again, in referring to the actions of nations or groups of people, I am also referring to individuals and their struggles with primordial emotions, which can enlist thought and behavior into maintaining and reinforcing the status quo of unresolved conflicts.

Path to Psychological Health

So what constitutes psychological health? In the following schema, I propose a different way of conceptualizing growth by using operational progressions consisting of six sequential steps: (1) acknowledging that a problem exists, (2) recognizing that solutions to the problem are available, (3) choosing the best solution, (4) implementing the chosen solution, (5) allowing feedback about the action chosen, and (6) re-engaging in the process, if necessary. Each of these steps will be described and are graphically represented in the following diagram:

Chart of Healthy Progression

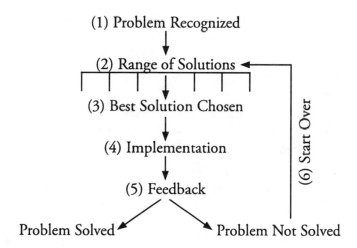

Figure 3-2 Chart of Healthy Progression

Step 1: Is a problem perceived? For example, some individuals blithely go along without ever knowing that they have a problem that needs to be addressed. An example is the boss who loses employees consistently but refuses to look at his own behavior to see if it is the cause. Others stubbornly refuse or are too apprehensive or disturbed to acknowledge that they have problems. "If I don't see the doctor, then I don't have cancer."

Step 2: Are the varieties of choices for solving the problem recognized? Is the problem approached with the feeling that there is no choice (the Child) even though the "only way" that was tried does not really work? "I know I lost everything at the gambling tables last time, but next time I'll be a winner."

Step 3: After recognizing an array of available choices for solving the problem, is there an ability to select the one that offers the best opportunity for an optimum solution? "It would be wise to apply for a promotion; it makes the most sense of all my choices."

Step 4: The problem is perceived, the range of choices are appreciated, and the best option is chosen. Can the choice be implemented? "When I apply for the promotion, am I willing to take on the new responsibilities or face the possibility of being turned down?"

Step 5: Feedback. This requires the willingness to evaluate whether or not the choice made and implemented resulted in the desired outcome. For example, the boss has just established meetings with employees. "I'm certain that my action was correct, so I need to acknowledge only that which verifies it."

This step confronts the individual with the uncomfortable possibility of having made the wrong choice—a difficult process. We are all inclined to believe that our assumptions are correct. After all, we would not have proceeded from false premises, right? This bias is not necessarily conscious and certainly not an overt attempt to be dishonest; it is simply a natural tendency. In science, the use of placebo-controlled, double-blind studies guards against our inclination to influence results to confirm our preconceptions. This means neither researcher nor subjects know if the administered substance is active or a placebo. Such study designs keep the researcher's prejudices and preconceptions from contaminating the outcome.

The appreciation that trial-and-error experiences enhance rather than diminish the self facilitates the acceptance of outcomes that differ from initial assumptions, making this fifth step easier to accomplish. Recall the previous story of Edison trying 10,000 times before his experiment succeeded. He was able to appreciate that those preliminary trials were of value in learning what did not work.

Step 6: Is there a willingness to start the whole process over again, realizing that something of considerable value has been gained in knowing what did not work and why? By repeating the cycle, we will eventually solve our problems and gain important insights in the process. Doing so, we appreciate feeling enhanced, not diminished, through the process of trial and error.

The examples used to illustrate these steps are simple ones, and people vary in their capacity to engage in all six steps in the numerous situations they encounter. Those situations that are most critical to optimum functioning in our families, work, and social relationships are the most important ones to measure. Paradoxically, the more peripheral the problems are to the emotional epicenter, the easier it is to fully engage the cycle from Step 1 to Step 6.

Most people find it hard to go beyond Step 4. Allowing oneself access to feedback may be painful and difficult if it is associated with the fear of being seen as wrong and, thereby, a lesser person. An elaborate process of rationalizations, distortions, and justifications may be used to support the correctness of the choice, regardless of the outcome. The might of denial is used to establish the right of action.

Getting past this block is vital to starting the process over in a more successful way. Using an example of a nation's actions to parallel that of an individual, think of the Vietnam War. Those in power in the United States had great hesitancy acknowledging mistaken choices, even refusing to do so. Secretary of State Robert McNamara spoke of the anguish that accompanied his belated reflections on the errors made.[13] Without feedback, no matter how painful, we cannot learn. Without learning, we cannot grow. History has yet to conclude the appropriateness of our nation's actions in Iraq. For nations, as for individuals, George Santayana's advice remains salient: "Those who do not learn from the past are condemned to repeat it."[14]

No Initial Mistakes

An important corollary regarding the actions we take and the decisions we make deserves special emphasis: Whatever a person does at any one time is exactly the right thing to do, in that person's mind, or he would not have chosen to engage in that specific behavior at that time. This may seem paradoxical and philosophically difficult to recognize. A simple example will illustrate the point.

It is the middle of the night and the streets are empty. You have stopped at a red light, which seems to take forever to change. Your bladder is full. The light does not change. No cars can be seen anywhere. You go through the red light, knowing that at this moment it is the right thing for you to do. Then you see the flashing red lights in your rearview mirror. New information you previously did not have is now available and tells you, "Not such a good idea after all."

Going through a red light when no one is around may be a simple, almost harmless, act compared with more profound behaviors. Can an evil act be similarly understood? Did Hitler do the right thing when he decided to exile and exterminate Jews, among whom were scientists, physicians, and scholars? Yes, *in his mind* he did. "If the dismissal of Jewish scientists means the annihilation of contemporary German science, then we shall do without science for a few years," Hitler said. In doing so, he closed the door on Germany's fifty-year record of world supremacy in science. Of the more than 1,500 refugees, including Einstein, Perutz, Haber, and Szilard, fifteen won Nobel Prizes. "Far from destroying the spirit of German scholarship, the Nazis had spread it all over the world."[15] Though Hitler was convinced of the correctness of his maniacal beliefs, it is difficult to imagine—if he had a sane moment—that he would have failed to realized how wrong he had been, based on what those exiled and killed could have contributed to a Nazi victory.

So it is with any action. A millisecond later, years later, or perhaps never, we may discern that what seemed to be right at the time was not really the best course to take. Only with the acquisition of new information can we look back and identify our errors. Mistakes are always judgments derived from retrospective evaluations, never prospective ones. With this in mind, we can appreciate that *when a sufficiently intelligent person does a dumb thing, it is for some significant reason.* That reason may not, as in Hitler's case, be one that makes sense to others, although there were, unfortunately, a large number of people who concurred with his madness in the belief that his reasoning was correct.

Retrospective vision is always 20/20. Prospective vision never can be. Many people decline the corrective lenses of feedback because the clarity might be perceived as "turning state's evidence" against the self. "If I was wrong then, I might be wrong now. Better not open that can of worms." For this reason the title of the aforementioned minister's sermon is so poignant: "What if I should awake before I die?"

Recriminations

To benefit from reflecting on past behaviors, we must avoid the trap of self-recrimination—"I was so dumb to have done that." Recriminations serve only to perpetuate problems, locking us in a self-negating loop. Establishing an environment of self-acceptance, self-reflection, and understanding enables us to grow. ("I am, after all, human, and humans do make mistakes"). Acceptance of the self while examining adverse behaviors is one of the keystone benefits in therapeutic relationships.

Fortunate is the child whose parents are able to clearly distinguish between his person and his behaviors, especially when those behaviors are undesirable. "I love you, but we must discuss your unacceptable behavior." We often hear the canard "unconditional love." There is no such thing. You either love, or you do not love, the person. This is separate from accepting or rejecting that person's behavior. A therapeutic ambience helps to foster this distinction, in contrast to a punitive or judgmental setting. For example, I sometimes say to patients regarding their conflicts, "If you want judgments, see an attorney. If you are looking for absolution, see a priest. If you are interested in understanding, then a therapist is the right person for you."

Los Angeles newspaper columnist Jack Smith began an article by writing, "My life is paved with the cobblestones of regrets."[16] All of us have those cobblestones. We ignore or refuse to acknowledge flashing red lights in life precisely because doing so means allowing feedback (Step 5) and having to question why we thought our original action or decision was best at the time. When we do allow ourselves that feedback, we can make different choices and gain from the benefit of our experiences. Cobblestones can serve as paving stones to a better future. But if change threatens our perception of stability or safety (the Child), we block feedback.

A humorous story comes to mind of a therapist who makes a clear, definitive statement about what the patient's struggles represent. The patient responds with an enthusiastic, "Aha, that's it! Why didn't you tell me this before?" The therapist sighs and replies, "I've been telling you this for the past five years." There is a crucial time when we are willing to recognize and be open to feedback from others or from ourselves. I coined a mantra to help me keep this in perspective: "There are none so deaf as those who will not *yet* hear, or so blind as those who will not *yet* see." Going forward with a sense of self-acceptance in an experientially informed and aware fashion is fundamental for emotional growth.

Authentic or Sincere?

The majority of our communications with other people can be viewed as *sincere*. However, authentic communication—unfortunately much less common—is ideally the goal to strive for, especially in our closest relationships. There is an important distinction between these words.

One derivation of the word sincere may be *sine cere,* meaning *without wax,* connoting an unadulterated purity of expression.[17] Supposedly Roman builders who did shoddy work would use stone-powder-impregnated wax between building blocks to make the seam look exactly fitted. I define *sincerity* as knowing beforehand the likely outcome of an action. Many of our actions are sincere. Consider an exchange between people passing in a hallway:

"How are you?"

"Fine."

"That's good."

This interaction is predictable and known by all. Just see what happens if in responding to the same question, one person says, "Terrible." The reply, "That's good," may still be the same. This is not because the questioner is uncaring or insincere. Rather, he is listening to a preprogrammed dialogue in his mind, which has always been perfunctorily the same, and not to the actual response.

By contrast, I consider *authenticity* to mean the inability to predict what the response will be. Sincere behavior is an important and totally appropriate social lubricant. But *authenticity of expression is the desirable goal in our closest relationships.* To be authentic means to be willing to tolerate an uncertain response, allow for the unpredictable, and really listen. We approach our significant relationships with unguarded intimacy when we cannot entirely predict the other persons' responses. There are no prerecordings in such interactions. Being uncertain of what will be said creates anxiety, and only when we are willing to tolerate this anxiety do we become authentic.

William Allen White commented, "I am not afraid of tomorrow, for I have seen yesterday, and love today."[18] In saying that he has seen yesterday, I believe he means that he has understood what was, as well as what was not, and has achieved peace about both. By "love," I believe he means being open and willing to experience the unpredictable with vulnerability—uncontaminated by fear of helplessness. This is, after all, the only way one can love.

In this chapter, I have laid the foundations of my theory by emphasizing our crucial need to bond as infants and to maintain the familiarity of those cues that signified survival. Earlier, I introduced the two terms used to describe two distinct states of being—Child and Adult—and described the differentiating characteristics defining each of these states.

We are now ready to approach the next chapter, which forms the crux of my thesis: Breaking free to grow from the Child to the Adult.

CHAPTER FOUR

Breaking Free

In order to thrive, we may have to give up what we once perceived as necessary to survive—another human paradox. Let me restate this truth in the terms I have presented: *In order to have what we Want, we have to give up what we Need.*

When our Needs are desirable cues, they become part of what we Want. I previously used the nightmarish reality of a concentration camp to illustrate a world turned upside down. The enormous effort required by the prisoners simply to survive in that environment, devoid of fundamental, decent Wants, is difficult to comprehend and we can readily empathize with those who felt like giving up.

How about when a person's world is right side up but his Need system still predominates over his Wants? Empathizing with a person whose actions diminish or destroy favorable circumstances and create or maintain painfully destructive conditions is much more difficult. How can we understand such behavior? Certainly, as much as it may seem otherwise, it is never based on the person's desire for misery. No one wants to be unhappy. Rather, turmoil results when antithetical and powerful Need cues from the past emotionally overwhelm what a person Wants in the present. Such individuals will snatch misery from the jaws of desire because they feel they must do so to survive.

A Linear Scale

Below is a linear scale, arbitrarily numbered, with zero in the center:

-5 __-4__ -3 __-2__ -1 _ [0]__ +1 _ +2__ +3 __+4__ +5

Needs   Wants

Figure 4-1

I ascribe to the negative numbers the adverse Needs from the past and to the positive numbers what is desired in real time. To move from adverse Needs (painful relationships, behaviors, feelings) to reach what we Want, we must traverse zero. The intellect says, "Go for it!" But the emotions say zero is fraught with loss, threat, and danger. Suddenly, we feel cautious and hesitant to move forward, because breaking free of what chains us to the past means giving up the familiar and predictable for the uncertain, the known for the unknown, the safe (even if painful) for the risky. When we are intensely immersed in conflict, reflected on the scale by a high negative number, zero does not look all that threatening. As the conflict lessens, we again approach zero, and it looms larger and more daunting.

The subtitle of this book—*How Chains from Childhood Keep Us from What We Want*—contains a play on the words *keep us* that, on the one hand, implies security and, on the other, restriction. Those chains are the Needs that keep us feeling safe with the familiar and predictable but also bind us to the past, preventing us from achieving what we Want.

An unfortunately common example that illustrates how solidly our chains can bind us in familiar but agonizing situations is the severely abused woman, hospitalized yet again for her injuries, who seems resolved this time to leave her abusive husband. Once more he is remorseful; he cries and begs her not to leave him. He promises, yet again, that this was the last time he will ever hurt her. Gradually his improving behavior diminishes the intensity of the wife's intolerable plight. On the linear scale, as the negative lessens, the relationship moves toward zero. With only some unpleasantness at times, neither of them is motivated to risk disrupting the marriage and make the fundamental changes that going through zero would entail. Feeling relatively so much better, the wife decides to stay with her husband. After all, she knows him and has a home, perhaps children, with him. She Wants a loving relationship, but who knows what would await her if she were to leave? Besides, things are not so bad now, are they?

The 1994 New Zealand movie *Once Were Warriors* depicts how incredibly powerful this compulsion to remain with the familiar can be. The wife tolerates repeated and severe beatings by the husband who afterward always expresses remorse, but the cycle continues. Only after their daughter's rape and suicide is the woman finally able to stop avoiding zero; she takes her children and leaves the husband. When the woman recognizes that the prospect of having no relationship is better than perpetuating a bad one, she reaches a turning point. Giving up the negative makes the positive possible.

The Exodus

Here is another example of how battle lines are drawn when what we Want conflicts with what we Need. Much can be learned about human psychology from the Bible. In this case, I am referring to the story of the Exodus. The retelling of the tale is the central theme of the Passover observation. Here was a tribe of Israelites[1] who, the myth relates, were sorely abused, oppressed, and enslaved by the Egyptian Pharaoh. Moses arises to lead them out of slavery and despair to the Promised Land—a land they desire and wish for but that, until now, had only been a dream. First, however, they must cross the desert. What happens? Many begin to complain and rebel. "What sort of leader are you?" they implore. "Why did you take us away from our homes? Yes, conditions were miserable, painful, and difficult, but we knew how to deal with them. We were surviving, had learned how to cope, and we knew what our losses would be. There was no uncertainty, no unpredictability. We were clearly far better off there than here, in this empty place, where we have nothing." Moses plaintively replies, "But just ahead lies what you have wanted all along." They retort, "How can we be sure? What we knew and had is better, although it was terrible, than what may or may not come to pass. There is too much uncertainty."

I have taken liberties with the dialogue, but the essence remains. The story goes on to describe how the Jews wandered for forty years to eliminate the generation that Needed slavery. This marvelous allegory illustrates how the path to the positive requires tolerating the emotional risk of traversing the zero of the barren desert—giving up the painful known past for the hoped-for but unknown future.

Those fortunate enough to have received the nurturing and support during childhood that enable them to explore the unknown with confidence (the gift parents can give by validating the child) may not find going through zero such an awesome task. For those whose lives are determined by Needs compatible with Wants, or those whose Wants transcend and supersede conflicting Needs, the journey beckons. In the book of Ruth (1:16), Ruth is willing to give up all that is familiar to her and travel into the unknown. Perhaps we could speculate that she had nurturing parents, or that she succeeded in having her Wants transcend her Needs, which allowed her to say, "Wherever you go, I shall go, wherever you live, I shall live."

A story is told of a psychoanalyst who survived World War II but lost everything familiar to him. After immigrating to New York, he established a successful practice, married, and had children. One day he decided to move to California. His friends marveled at the ease with which he could, once again, subject himself to being uprooted. Although this time it was his choice, friends commented that he must have had a fantastic therapist to be able to forfeit all his security and face the unknown. "Yes," he replied, "It was Adolf Hitler." Of course, what he meant was that the horrible circumstances imposed on him by the war allowed him to master any fears about change and uncertainty.

Does Change Take Time?

The Passover allegory conveys the idea that the Hebrews needed forty years of wandering to prepare for their new identity as a free people. I do not want to endorse the notion implied in the story that change takes a long time. I am inclined to believe that change is an instant thing—not unlike falling off the edge of a cliff. How long does it take to fall? Not very long. What does take time, however, is getting to the edge, teetering there, and then risking stepping forward. I like the analogy of the cliff because it represents both the challenge and the threat of change. It symbolically portrays all the ideas discussed earlier regarding vulnerability versus helplessness, uncertainty, threat to survival, and the loss of familiar ground that was deemed safe.

Richard Rabkin proposes that perhaps for some, therapy is a face-saving ritual that allows a person to change.[2] After all, how does one who behaves in a destructive fashion suddenly announce that he will be different? If it results from therapy, the transition can occur in a socially approved way.

That person can now be different without others questioning why he did not change earlier. The philosophical question Rabkin raises—whether the unconscious is a necessary construct—is an interesting one, though it does not necessarily negate the existence of unconscious conflicts.

Freud postulated that successfully mastering a traumatic situation might be the equivalent of an analysis.[3] By way of an analogy to what he inferred, imagine the captain of a ship caught in a terrible storm. The waves are mountainous, and the ship is in great danger. To survive, he must eliminate all the excessive and unnecessary baggage that weighs down the ship. He must evaluate everything on board and determine what is necessary and what is burdensome. In the process of therapy, or growth of any sort, we must similarly examine and risk discarding what we conclude to be excess emotional baggage. All the old cargo from the past that is not of value in the present must go. The process is one of recognizing, evaluating, and discarding. Because we cannot jettison our pasts, discarding here means decommissioning the old ways. The ship not only stays afloat but can now sail to new ports.

Continuing with the nautical metaphor, each of us resembles a boat whose anchor, representing our unresolved past, hangs overboard in the unseen depths. Despite the throttle being thrown wide open, the boat can muster only limited forward movement because of the anchor's drag. Just as the anchor is an integral part of the boat, we cannot simply cut the line, any more than we can eliminate our own past, a vital component to our being. Raising the anchor, which symbolizes previously unseen conflicts that we are now able to bring on board, eliminates the drag. Once we do so and the boat is freed, we can fully dedicate our efforts to moving ahead. Patients have likened this experience to that of the motorboat operator who has lifted his anchor. A burst of creative energy, previously unavailable, empowers the person and propels him forward toward new ventures. Illuminating the past brightens the future.

In Genesis 35:10, Jacob encounters an angel with whom he wrestles, and in the process, he is transformed into Israel. I take this to be an allegory of facing one's conflicts, engaging them, and emerging successfully and remarkably changed. William James, in a late nineteenth century work, collected stories of people whose lives were dramatically changed as the result of some significant event.[4] These transformational encounters exemplify the relative immediacy of change when the circumstances are sufficiently poignant and the individual is ready.

I have emphasized the importance of preparing for change in order for change to occur. A Zen expression says that when the pupil is ready, the teacher appears. I believe that where learning lives, teachers abound. Through whatever aegis, once we welcome change, it is not a lengthy process. Growth, however, is a life-long adventure.

Change Reflects Empowerment

Freud asserted that change depends on the relationship between pain and fear. If the pain associated with the old increases and/or the fear of the new decreases, we will change.[5] For example, a person who suffers from agoraphobia and for years confines himself to one room of his home could quickly be "cured." Should the house catch fire, he would feel significantly less reticent about going outside. Although I certainly do not recommend this approach, some dramatic therapies for phobias, such as immersion and exposure, can be highly effective.

Another important dimension to what makes change feasible, discussed at length previously, warrants repetition: *Change would be impossible if the childhood perception of vulnerability as synonymous with helplessness were true in adulthood.* It is exactly because the two perceptions no longer equate that one can risk change.

Reasonable chances can be taken by the **A**dult who knows that if something does not work out he would still have learned and gained from the experience. There may be delay and disappointment—perhaps even pain—in reaching the coveted goal, but not the devastation of being rendered helpless. The antidote to the corrosive poison of feeling helpless is allowing oneself to be vulnerable whenever appropriate and recognizing that choices always exist. The ability to exercise those options that will engender life improvement empowers us and enables us to travel to once only wished-for and dreamed-of places.

Repression, Suppression, and Sublimation

We employ two defense mechanisms—*repression* (unconscious forgetting) and *suppression* (conscious or preconscious forgetting)—in attempting to deny that distressing perceptions and feelings play a significant role in our lives. It is a trick we perpetrate on ourselves. We use these mechanisms to store our pain, like nuclear waste, in the deepest crevices of our beings. But the radioactivity impinges on our daily lives. As in the example of the boat's anchor, unresolved conflicts must be acknowledged, identified, brought on board, and dealt with in order to neutralize the power that Needs wield.

Some people's antipathy toward therapy may arise from their fear of having to acknowledge forces within themselves of which they were previously unaware and that these forces decisively influence and even determine their behavior. It is an unpalatable medicine to have to swallow. Rationalizing our behavior seems so much easier than exploring unconsidered forces. The Gospel according to John (8:31-36) urges, "The truth shall make you free," and Akenside counsels, "Where Truth deigns to come, Her sister Liberty will not be far."[6]

Sublimation is another defense mechanism which we use to handle conflicts without our full awareness. Although we may not address the conflicts directly, we displace—sublimate—them into acceptable and constructive outlets, which are often valued and even desired by society. For example, the little boy who gets a thrill out of cutting up bugs because he needs to be in control and so avoid his own fearful feelings may become a successful surgeon in adulthood without ever addressing the underlying emotions. The **Adult** successfully reins in the **Child**. People who sublimate unresolved issues generally do not seek therapy unless the sublimation fails to contain the conflict.

It is very difficult to see oneself fully—particularly those aspects of the self that contain significantly painful conflict, no matter how clearly others may see them. Eric Berne once interviewed a troubled family of four. The mother had brought Berne's book *Games People Play*[7] and asked him to autograph it. She thanked him for the insights he presented which made it possible for her to identify everyone's game. She could now easily give a name to the conflicts acted out by all those whom she encountered, she said. Without delay Berne replied, "Yes, except perhaps your own!"[8] Grotstein has similarly commented, "The trouble with self-analysis lies in the counter-transference."[9]

Talking Out or Acting Out

Imagine a device with two hydraulic cylinders. One is labeled *feelings* and the other *behavior*. Pushing down on one simply causes the other to rise up. That device symbolizes us. When we push down significant feelings through repression or suppression, we do not eliminate them. Instead, those feelings will pop right back up in the form of symptomatic behavior. A very simple illustration is that of a man who says he is totally free of any feelings of prejudice. Nevertheless, he zealously avoids dealing with any member of minority groups. Having repressed his undesirable feelings, he acts them out through his behavior. Behavior thus becomes employed to express what is denied emotionally.

By developing physical symptoms, we have another outlet besides behavior for releasing our unacknowledged significant feelings. Perhaps a third cylinder on the above device could be labeled *somatization*. It was a common expression of unresolved inner turmoil in Freud's day when a patient might present with symptoms of overt paralysis, generalized body weakness, or vague aches and pains that had no physical cause.

The following is a dramatic example of physical symptoms representing emotional conflict. A family, consisting of parents and their teenage daughter, sought therapy because of concerns about the daughter's emotional withdrawal. It quickly became clear that the father and daughter acted as if controlled by the threat that the mother's intestinal symptoms might flare up were she to become upset. This created an emotional tyranny in the family. If something was said with which the mother disagreed, she would suddenly get painful cramps and rectal bleeding, necessitating a trip to the hospital. The mother employed physical symptoms to control her own unacknowledged childhood fears, thereby indirectly expressing through her behavior what she was unable to verbalize. She feared that her present family would gang up on her and render her helpless, as had happened to her in childhood. Now the mother's behavior made the father and daughter the helpless ones. Paradoxically, the mother was always on the verge of being rendered helpless herself by the very method she employed to solve her childhood trauma. The control she supposedly wielded served only to perpetuate her fears and her past.

An even more stunning example of emotional conflict expressed through physical symptoms is the case of a mother, a father, and their two sons who were seen in a family therapy session.[10] One son, the identified patient, had been hospitalized because of psychotic symptoms. During the session, conflict between the parents that had never before been openly expressed was directly, if very subtly voiced, which shifted the focus away from the hospitalized son, a marked deviation from the family's ordinary communication pattern. The ever-so-slight change did not seem either significant or dramatic to the therapist, who would have offered greater support if the profundity of the shift had been recognized.

During the following week, the hospitalized son's condition worsened, the father suffered a heart attack, the mother was hospitalized for gall bladder pain, and the other son, whose driving record had been excellent, rear-ended a vehicle and destroyed his own car. Coincidence? Hardly. The family recoiled from acknowledging the chronic, distressing feelings between the parents as though touching a hot stove. Behavior and symptoms replaced any direct recognition of emotional distress. Clearly more intensive support was necessary than was initially evident. This case dramatically demonstrates how the family shunted emotional expressions into both physical symptoms and behavior.

No matter what a person in the present may wish, he must resolve his conflicted behaviors—which are fueled by early survival-oriented perceptions—before he can attain his yearned-for goals. All therapies are ultimately oriented toward this resolution, although not all will directly address the underlying perceptions. This will be discussed more fully in the chapters on psychotherapy. Whatever their theoretical orientation, all therapists aspire to support their patients in reaching the other side of zero as they break free of the past and grow in the present.

The more we try to deny traumatic or problematic past experiences, the more we trap ourselves in perpetuating our painful perceptions from our childhood. In adulthood, we recapitulate significant unresolved mind-sets, such as being abused, disregarded, or disrespected as children. A corollary of behavioral manifestations of feelings is using verbalizations to *avoid* expressing feelings: that is, a person talks endlessly about anything and everything except that which is emotionally significant to him. Whatever the mechanism employed, pushing down the "feelings cylinder" results in past conflicts being perpetuated in the present through the popping up of behavior. It is akin to using a do-it-yourself crucifixion kit and then anguishing over the pain suffered.

I have suggested a very different view of the often-touted idea of healing the inner child. The only possible resolution of childhood conflicts is for the **A**dult to acknowledge and accept the experiences that were the child's. This means knowing that the past cannot be other than what it was. We can change our *feelings* about the past, but we cannot change the *events* of the past. With this awareness there comes a modicum of healing. However, if by *healing* we mean creating a new childhood, then no healing is possible—we must let go of the past. Breaking free and risking going through zero represents this concept: the path to becoming an **A**dult.

Symbolically, the past is the place where we used to live but do not anymore. The popular notion that "it is never too late to have a good childhood" is nonsensical. *It is never too late to have a satisfying adulthood,* however. As adults, we must recognize that what we missed as children we cannot replace in the present, which inevitably leaves a hole. Paradoxically, accepting that there is a hole and understanding why allows one to become whole and fulfilled.

The Blame Game Cop-Out

Some adult children blame or attack their parent(s) for what was missing in their childhoods. Such anger or resentment testifies to the lack of conflict resolution and is an exercise in futility. For one thing, the present parents bear only a faint resemblance to the childhood parents, just as the current adult offspring bears only a faint resemblance to the child he once was. Expressing anger at the parents simply reinforces the feelings of helplessness from childhood, which perpetuates in the adult the Child state as he acts as though he still Needs the parents' validation. A passively abused or neglected child, though angry, is still a child.

Picture two kids at the bottom of a deep pit. One silently endures while the other rages. Neither one is aware of being anywhere other than in the pit. Blaming parents for past deeds only impedes and delays resolution of the conflict, as though the adult is still in the pit. It also denies the healing realization that our parents were once children themselves and that they learned to parent from their own parents. We can go back generation upon generation and see unresolved problems getting passed along through either passive compliance or angry rebellion. Both represent two sides of the same coin: feeling trapped by what was and ignoring what could be. The "buck" of conflict either stops here and now or gets passed on to the next generation.

Ralph Greenson gave a talk entitled "Mrs. Portnoy Answers Back," a response structured around Philip Roth's book *Portnoy's Complaint*. In his presentation, Greenson had Mrs. Portnoy say, "Alex, I did what I thought was best. I may have made mistakes and can look back now and maybe wish I had done things differently. But, I am no longer the mother to a little boy. If something is missing, it is up to you to get it for yourself now and stop blaming me."[11] Good advice!

In the same vein, Jean-Paul Sartre observed, "We are what we make of what others have made of us."[12] This implies being willing to give up trying to redo the past and taking the best possible care of oneself in the present. Emotionally fearful of this, some will counter, "But if I give up trying to get cared for as a kid, then I won't ever be cared for." This is yet another example of the awesome challenge involved in journeying through zero.

The more a person values himself in a meaningful way, the more he has to offer a companion who in turn will be someone who also has a sense of self-worth and the capacity for sharing, since we choose partners who are at about the same level of maturity as we ourselves are.[13] By actualizing the growth from our primary state of immature dependence (Child) to a state of autonomy and mature dependence (Adult), we best prepare ourselves for the real experience of love. This contradicts the notion that being grown up and able to take care of oneself means losing the chance to be cared for. The desire to have the best possible mate becomes realized by being the best possible person. This requires that we take responsibility for ourselves and not blame others for our problems.

When Then Is Now and Here Is There

The child's solutions to conflicts (then) often become the adult's problems (now). The child who in the face of deprivation withdraws and denies having any desires has arrived at a good solution for dealing with his pain, given the lack of available options. Without desires, he is freed from the emotional distress caused by the futility of longing for what he cannot have. But if this carries over to adulthood, the solution of denying desires now becomes the problem that perpetuates feeling deprived. What worked well when there were no choices if continued obviates the awareness that choices exist. Deprivation was a reality foisted on the child who subsequently artificially imposes it on himself—in the Child state. It therefore becomes the cue to the familiarity of home and in adulthood is expected in intimate relationships.

Similarly, what is good for the adult (and leads to being an Adult) is likely experienced as bad for the Child, because the Child is threatened with the loss of the familiar—of having to leave home. The adult, however, must let go of what he Needed and move on if he is to become an autonomous Adult. Zero looms ever larger. Recall the man's dream of seeing the child he once was lying in the gutter. Instead of facing the necessary but distressing task of accepting what once was and moving on, a person may try to deny that he has unresolved problems—refusing to hear the chains rattling. As a result, the conflicts are perpetuated rather than being resolved.

The adult faces the daunting task of having to accept that no amount of effort spent in the present will make the past other than what it was. Trying to change history and achieve some denied goal of the child is impossible. The emotional hunger to change the past may fuel great efforts in the present, but those efforts will be futile. A person may have major accomplishments—achievements acknowledged by others—yet feel as empty and devoid of value as he did as a child. Just look at the lonely, isolated, or depressed CEO, professor, movie star, businessman, *et al*. To the outside world, he looks incredibly successful, yet he may consider himself to be unfulfilled, a failure.

I found one particular vignette of *Sesame Street* fascinating. One puppet character said to the other, "Come over here."

"I am here," replied the other.

"No, you are there. I am here."

"Oh no, I am the one who is here, and it is you who are there." While watching this exchange, I was struck by how often people start "here," feeling they are not okay, and then believe they will be okay once they get to "there." Of course when they get "there," they are once again "here" and still feel invalid, regardless of any significant external achievements.

Does this mean that striving for fulfillment is futile? Not at all. It is not the striving that is the problem. We may hope to change past unworthy *then*-feelings solely through some present, external *now*-accomplishment, but we will never succeed in doing so. The *Sesame Street* segment poignantly demonstrates that unless the journey starts with valid feelings of one's own unique worth, it does not matter where one travels. Start "here" feeling not okay, and you get wherever "there" may be feeling not okay. The player who is convinced that he has three strikes against him before coming to bat experiences hitting the ball out of the park as avoiding being exposed as a failure, at least until the next time at bat, rather than as a success.

Being and Doing

Our society often focuses its attention on what we do (our occupations) and significantly less on how we feel (our beings). In what follows, I point out an important aspect of both issues in the hope that the question of feeling can be appreciated as being at least as important as that of doing.

Irving Yalom, a professor of psychiatry at Stanford University, described an informal survey he took among students in a medical school class.[14] He asked them to anonymously write their deepest secret fears on pieces of paper, fold them, and turn them in. Amazingly, a large number of this very academically accomplished group wrote that they feared they were inadequate. From their external achievements, one would expect them to feel good about themselves. It is remarkable how many people are apprehensive about being "busted by the fraud squad." How come? It may be because how they feel about themselves as beings differs from how they feel about what they do—their accomplishments or professions.

Often we view achievements not as intrinsically valuable but as a necessary prelude to whatever the next step may be. It is the next step that will count! Kindergarten exists to get to the first grade, middle school to get to high school, and so forth. The concept of stopping long enough to "smell the roses," though trite, speaks to the importance of valuing whatever we experience at the moment. Culturally we are trained to focus on our occupations as statements of our worth. The two questions most often asked of us when we meet someone new are "What is your name?" and "What do you do?" It is as though we know the worth of the person by the answers to these questions.

Occasionally, if feeling mischievous, I will answer the question "What do you do?" by saying, "The best I possibly can at any given moment, and it isn't easy." This tends to disorient the questioner who is looking for a reply that fits into a vocational category. When he subsequently learns that I am a psychiatrist, he may nod patronizingly, as though he is now able to attribute my bizarre nonresponse. So ingrained is our assumption that vocation equals value that the potential profundity of the actual reply is completely lost.

In the 1970s, when cults were on the rise and the focus of a great deal of attention, there was considerable concern about the "cream" of young adults being caught up in such organizations. A group of Jewish and Christian leaders studied the phenomenon. Their findings were striking and simply stated. When young people come to churches or synagogues they are asked, "What is your name and what do you do?" or "What are you going to do?" The cults, on the other hand, ask, "What is your name and how are you feeling?" That was enough to create a "vacuum cleaner" effect: These kids got sucked up into what, unfortunately, was often a nefarious undertaking because they thought the cults cared about how they were, not what they would achieve. These were not just troubled youngsters but included healthy, mentally stable adolescents and young adults. The results emphasized the importance of focusing not just on what people do but also on how they feel. Remember the simple study that showed that we experience love through understanding. The feelings of attunement and connectedness induced when we are asked "How do you feel?" comes from its focus on our being, not just our doing.

I certainly am not ignoring the importance of doing and of accomplishments, especially in our culture. At the least, I want to emphasize the equal importance of the person as a being. Clearly our emotional struggles for self-value emerge from the recognition of ourselves as beings. It would be foolish to suggest that a great sense of value cannot also come from what we do. Of course it can—but there must be a space available within us for affirmation that is uncontaminated by self-negation. If we start with "I'm okay as a person," then we can value and incorporate the gratification we gain from our accomplishments. Although there may be other ways to develop self-regard, I am stressing breaking free from the distressing, limiting, familiar chains of the Child and then tolerating the journey through zero to the autonomy of the Adult.

Many people spend lives of quiet desperation on an emotional treadmill. Picture a person on such a treadmill who no matter how fast or hard he runs remains in the same place. For all his effort, he never gets ahead; the exertion simply keeps him from falling back. Now add to this image a monster lurking with open jaws at the back end of the treadmill. The fearsome beast represents whatever in the past was feared or distressing. If stopping truly meant being devoured, how could the person possibly stop running? Yet stopping would mean that the momentum would carry the runner back—to the open jaws of self-negation.

Here is another paradox of this situation: The desperate adult runner feeds the monster only by conferring on it the same power he felt it had when he was a child. After all, why else would he be running? The beast devours with gusto those present behaviors that are commandeered to express unacknowledged past feelings. No matter how much the person runs—how much he does, how much he accomplishes—he will never get away from the beast. Avoiding confronting whatever the fears from the past may be serves to perpetuate the conflicts that grow ever larger in the present. The runner only feels drained of energy, and the monster only gets fatter!

The Paradox of Conflict

Paradoxically, internal conflict always paints us into the very corner we are desperately trying to avoid. Recall the earlier metaphor of the hydraulic cylinder device. Pushing down feelings through repression or suppression naturally results in the acting out (popping up) of these feelings. We often behave like the traveler in the story who was told that death awaited him in the next town. Rather than face the fears of his own mortality, he immediately changed his destination, only to discover that he had confused the places and thus arrived in the very city from which he was trying to escape. This is also the moral of Sophocles's play "Oedipus Rex." It tells of the prophecy that Oedipus will kill his father, Laius, and father children with his mother, Jocasta. To prevent this, Jocasta abandons the infant Oedipus to die in the mountains, but another royal family rescues and takes him in. He grows up and fulfills the dire predictions of his fate.

Without resorting to any theosophical considerations, I suggest that this is a kind of predestination—the predestination of an emotionally determined fate of endlessly repeating unresolved past conflicts. We dread and wish to escape from having to deal with painful issues, yet we desperately cling to these chains of the past. Buddhist reincarnation philosophy is very clear: What is not dealt with in this life must be faced in the next. We can translate this to mean that what is not dealt with today will simply lurk, awaiting tomorrow. Resolving conflicts requires facing—and not shunning—whatever fears we may have.

Picture the usual image of a child awakening at night in fear of the monster in the closet. The parent tries to comfort and reassure him by turning on the light and opening the closet door. Fear is faced. Metaphorically, if an adult keeps the door shut on his Child fears, he believes he has avoided the danger of whatever lurks behind the closed door. With the door closed he paradoxically fancies himself free of his terror, except he dares not leave the room lest the demons emerge in his absence. This obviously limits how far he can emotionally travel in his life. This is the pseudo-adult state. The symbolic profundity of undertaking the journey that beckons when fears are faced is perhaps expressed by the powerful imagery in Psalm 23: "The Lord is my shepherd; I shall not want. He makes me lie down in green pastures, and leads me besides the still waters. Yea, *though I walk through the valley of the shadow of death I will fear no evil, for thou art with me.*" For those who do not subscribe to an anthropomorphic image of God, the guiding shepherd image is a good representation of the Adult self.

When a person declines to participate in conflicted patterns of behavior with others, he acknowledges that it is impossible to change what was, no matter how often it is restaged and no matter with whom it is attempted. He can change his feelings about what has happened, but he cannot change the events themselves. The attempt is a lost endeavor. *The only way to win a game called "you lose" is not to play.* The only way not to play is to change today instead of trying to change yesterday.

Although we may restage old losing games in any of our interactions with others, we do so particularly in our most emotionally intimate relationships with our mates and families. For this reason, in the next chapter, I focus on how we go about selecting our mates and the interactions (Needs) that interfere with fulfillment (Wants) in our relationships.

CHAPTER FIVE

_____

Choosing our Mates

Marriages are not made in heaven; they are made in childhood. In choosing mates, we try to avoid letting go of the chains from childhood and thereby never have to go through zero. If the Child within us can find the Child in a prospective mate who knows exactly what home means to both of us, then the kids never have to leave home—never have to confront zero. Although I certainly acknowledge that many researchers have presented a variety of theories about mate selection, I intend to focus on this one salient theme and refer readers to a review of the literature cited for a discussion of others.[1]

As children, we learn from parents and family what role we are to play in life and in relationships with others. Like the child in medieval times whose traveling minstrel family put on the same play in every town, we learn everyone's part by heart through constant repetition. We may hate the play, despise the characters, or loathe the ending, but it becomes a part of us. It is, after all, "the only play in town." Much as we may wish for a comedy and not a tragedy, as adults we just cast new leads in the same old play if we stay tethered to the familiarity of the Child's Needs. No matter how many new lead actors may play the title role, Shakespeare's _Hamlet_ still remains a tragedy when the curtain falls. Only if and when the script changes will the play end differently.

Children learn under the powerful reality of having no choice, which leads to idealization, as I discussed earlier. It is this idealized optionlessness that is central to the development of a child's Needs and which becomes incorporated in the **Child** part of the adult as the core element in adult conflict development. Whether male or female, we incorporate three major roles that broadly encompass what we perceive as our function in relationships and what we expect the roles of our partners to be. These roles and relationships apply *regardless of what the couple's sexual orientation may be;* and the characteristics of the roles are not biologically defined, aside from the nuances of human reproduction and suckling at the breast.

Context	Male	Female
In the World	Man	Woman
In Marriage	Husband	Wife
As Parents	Father	Mother

Figure 5-1 Six Marital Roles

During childhood this model becomes incorporated into our sense of place and person. The way our families define and model these roles forms the Need system that cues us to being home and feeling connected. As emphasized previously, Needs are not inherently good or bad—they just are. Those that we desire as adults we incorporate into Wants. My focus, however, is on the aspects of the Needs that lead to conflict in adulthood because they contradict what we Want.

When we were children these early cues signaled safety, even if they were painful and dangerous. We always perceived them as better than having nothing, since without our families, no matter how imperfect they were, we could not have survived. The classic needlepoint sampler reads, "Be it ever so humble, there is no place like home." If, however, what we desire as adults is beyond reach of the **Child's** Needs, the sampler more accurately would read, "Be it ever so miserable, there is no place like home."

Again, no one wants to be unhappy. But if the cues that define home for us are painful and we pursue those cues in new relationships, we are bound to be as unhappy as we were as children. The **Child's** conflicted Needs are then contrary to what the **Adult** Wants. In trying to help patients understand the forces within them that contribute to their mutual collusion in conflicts and create their unhappiness, I may state, "I understand that you don't want the problems to continue, and that you're upset by your partner's or your own behavior. Let's focus on why a part of you may Need exactly what you don't Want." I am asking the patient to begin to recognize the price he is paying for the "soothing sound" of his rattling chains.

Moth to Flame

A person who endeavors to maintain Need cues on behalf of his **Child** in order to avoid confronting his fear of change incurs inordinate emotional costs as an adult. This constitutes emotional usury which continues to be paid until his conflicts are resolved and his **Adult** emerges. "This is easier said than done" is, in this case, a major understatement! On his thirtieth anniversary broadcast, Garrison Keillor commented that marriage is "God's way for people to avoid having to fight with strangers." If this seems cynical, it is not. Even a cursory view of divorce statistics reveals the toll taken by unresolved conflicted Needs and how often these conflicts re-emerge in each subsequent relationship. Not unlike the moth drawn to the flame, there may be a powerful, compelling force drawing one person to another that does not bode well. The fact that the vast majority of those who divorce will remarry reinforces the idea that human beings are social animals seeking intimate connections. It also implies that the problem is not with the institution of marriage but rather with the inmates of the institution.

We do not marry strangers. We look for partners who have the same thematic chains—that is, the same Need systems that we have. Yes, at times it appears that "love is blind" or that "opposites attract," but "birds of a feather flock together" more accurately defines human attraction. Apropos of that latter aphorism, Jared Diamond describes how powerfully people are attracted to those who look just like them[2]. Several other studies demonstrate the validity of this observation.[3] Given that we usually resemble our families, this makes sense. The attraction becomes magnetic for the familiar/familial. (Note the remarkable similarity of those two words. Of course, both stem from the same root, and therefore the most familiar is going to be that which is the most familial. I will continue to use this conjunction of words to emphasize the psychological connection of the familiar [recognizable, frequently seen or experienced] and the familial [related to the family].)

To get a glimmer of the power of this attraction, think of being in a foreign country and not speaking the language. Everything and everyone seems strange and somewhat distant because of the language barrier. Suddenly you hear a person speaking your native tongue. You feel a compelling desire to meet that person and relate to him.

Though I use language as metaphor to illustrate the attraction certain people exert on us, I have actually had the opportunity to work with couples in which one person did not initially speak English, such as embassy officials and military personnel who met their mates while stationed overseas. When the foreign partner learned English and problems arose in the marriage for which they sought help, the matching themes of what intimate relationships mean in their respective families of origin astounded me. Although not speaking the same language when they met, they shared a profound nonverbal communication of familiarity.

The Need systems reflecting the Child part of each person in a relationship fit like a key in a lock. Together the partners replay familial themes and patterns. In my clinical experience, I have found substantiation for this interlocking in every couple I have worked with, so much so that I acknowledge that this is my orientation when working with couples.[4] Americans tend to view arranged marriages with disdain. The thought of it repels us. Yet the scripts we get from our parents ultimately arrange ours.

It's Just with Him/Her

People often comment that they do not have problems with anybody else but their spouses. "Of all the guys I've dated, I never had the difficulty that I have with you," a wife proclaims. That is all well and good to say. The fact is that she chose not to marry the people with whom she got along. Women may say that they can speak to and be understood by everyone else except their husbands. Some men allude to having had no difficulty with feelings of sexual inadequacy with other women, but with their wives they are impotent. They fail to appreciate that we are always most conflicted with the very people to whom we are the closest. Who else would it be if not our most emotionally intimate partners?

Major unresolved issues commonly manifest themselves in our marital relationships. However, continuing conflict requires that both partners collude in maintaining the problems rather than solving them. Such relationships may be deep and meaningful, but in the troubled areas the partners compromise what each of them desires in order to avoid "rocking the boat." The greater the emotional distance from the epicenter of unresolved issues a couple maintains, the more contented they may appear—a contentedness paid for by accepting superficiality. Either or both may seek a deeper sense of satisfaction through some emotional investment outside the marriage, such as an affair with work, hobbies, sports, or another person. The participant sees the affair as an environment in which he can let down his defenses and experience a closeness not found with his mate. The closeness is only an illusion, made possible because the issues he has with his spouse do not exist in the affair—that is, unless those who participate in the affair marry.

Casual relationships with others provide only time-outs from conflicts, not resolutions. Such relationships can be likened to playing pro ball on a sandlot. The home runs do not mean that much. The problems emerge when moving back into the major leagues. Another kind of time-out may occur with couples on vacation, when they can communicate easily and comfortably with their spouses—until returning home. Couples may have very gratifying experiences in circumstances when their unexplored conflicts are not being activated, similar to performers who can be intimate with their anonymous audiences but not with their spouses or children. In such situations, the **Child** may be "sleeping," but the **Adult** is also absent.

Of course, individuals who marry are very different from one another in many ways. But it is not their dissimilarities that precipitate problems. To the contrary, they ensue from the shared sameness of their converging Needs, which complement each partner's internal sense of "being home"—even if that is the last place either one of them would Want to be.

Because of these shared Needs, *couples are emotional twins.* As a simple example, consider John and Mary's relationship. John is "hail fellow well met," outgoing, jovial, and adventuresome. Mary is quiet, reserved, and hesitant in social situations. Friends comment that surely love is blind. "What could they possibly see in each other?" It is their sameness that attracted them to each other; they share the same underlying fundamental perception that the world is a dangerous place. John deals with his fears by being counterphobic, while Mary behaviorally expresses hers directly. The other's way of dealing with the same problem may also intrigue the partners. This sameness gives rise to both the hope in and the frustration of relationships—two edges of the shared sword.

Both John and Mary could potentially understand, better than most others, the pain arising from the essence of the shared meaning of their childhood experiences. Since they grew up in psychologically similar environments, they are uniquely able to help each other resolve their shared conflicts, if they so desire. The fly in the ointment is that they also share the same Need system with the interlocking sense of self, others, relationships, and the world. They can—and do—easily collude in perpetuating the old problems. This is the other edge of the sword that cuts. Whenever a couple's shared **Child Needs** predominate over **Adult Wants**, predictably they perpetuate their conflicts.

The Dangerous, Desired Familiar

Thus we seek partners with whom we can collude in recapitulating unresolved issues from the past. This usually unconscious component— the ability to restage mutual childhood conflicts in the relationship— ultimately determines our choice of mates. Certainly many other factors in our conscious awareness also draw us to our partners. When asked what we think attracted us to one another, we easily enumerate those latter, acknowledged, and desirable characteristics. But these are not the source of the potential problems. Rather those will arise from our partner's familiar way of rattling chains that captivated us in the first place, even if we are unaware of the sound.

I tell patients who begin to date, especially those re-entering the dating arena after a divorce, that finding someone compellingly alluring calls for cautious awareness. Going slowly at this juncture when objective awareness is most important is not easy, because wonderful feelings of being in love may obscure reason. Again we are drawn to people who share our Need system with the consequent potential for recreating unresolved primary conflicts in the relationship. A divorced person who has not resolved prior problems may have struggled to get out of the frying pan only to end up in the fire by repeating the old conflicts in a new relationship. The urge to merge may require a swerve for the relationship to be successful. The psychoanalytic researcher Robert Stoller, in discussing what ultimately stimulates powerfully erotic feelings, said rather succinctly that "we are drawn to new battlefields upon which old battles are waged, hoping to be victorious—this time."[5]

When we find a person alluring, the attraction, per se, is not the problem. That is a delightful feeling, powerfully reinforced by chemicals, especially the neurotransmitter dopamine (which also reinforces addiction). The concern must focus on the degree to which *both* partners recognize the mutual influence of their shared past Needs. Falling in love at first sight often sets the stage for an old play's rerun. It surprises most people in love that they, unlike people whose relationships develop gradually, must work more diligently at resolving the old in order to have the new. The gradually developing partnerships may grow more lovingly intimate over time because the pair are starting out at a neutral point. It follows from this that giving a person who does not necessarily attract—but at least does not repel—us a chance may lead to a truly different relationship.

Any relationship's success depends on a shared commitment to the resolution rather than the perpetuation of conflicts. Some people deal with difficulties by projecting them onto their partners—in essence saying, "The trouble with me is you." For those people, the following corollary, mentioned previously, may be both difficult and sobering to accept: We are drawn to intimate partners who have about the same degree of emotional maturity as we have.[6] Much like water finds its own level, we find our own developmental level in our intimate relationships. In addition, both partners bear equal responsibility for their relationship's troubles, as well as for the resolution of those troubles.

Finding Our Equal Fragment

How do we go about finding our partners? The answer lies in the power of nonverbal communication. It goes back to King Frederick II's question—what is our primary language? It is, of course, the nonverbal. Through the phenomenal power of this nonverbal language, we find partners who share our Need systems.

If the Child within us can find a partner whose Need system corresponds to ours, then the Child never has to leave home. If we never have to leave home, we never have to break free and confront zero. The few individuals whose Needs are in complete accord with their Wants run on autopilot in the selection of their mates and in the conduct of their lives. The old song lyric, "Some enchanted evening, you will see a stranger across a crowded room, and suddenly you will know," reflects the power of this nonverbal communication. However, the (modified) lyric, "I Need a girl/guy just like the girl/guy who married dear old mom/dad," much better characterizes the "stranger." If we dislike our parents' relationship, we sometimes play a trick on ourselves by choosing a mate who seems to be the exact opposite of our parental model. The parental opposite simply parades as the reverse of the same coin, as I will later describe in detail.

Carl Witaker, a pioneering family therapist, succinctly captured the ideas I present in this chapter in one of his relationship seminars. At the time, statistics showed a dramatic increase in the divorce rate. Someone asked Witaker what he thought about this escalation. With an incredible sense of comedic timing, he answered, "I don't believe in divorce." A murmur echoed across the audience of therapists, half of whom were probably divorced. Continuing after a pregnant pause, he said, "For that matter, I don't believe in marriage." This really baffled the group. Then came the punch line, "I don't believe in people. *I think we are all just fragments of our families that they sent out to reproduce themselves!*"[7]

This notion of finding the equal fragment in a mate yields a crucial correlate. *Conflicts in relationships are fifty-fifty propositions.* That is, each partner has a 50 percent responsibility for perpetuating and resolving the relationship's problems. There is no good or bad guy in a marriage. To illustrate this mutuality, picture two people dancing together—say, Fred Astaire and Ginger Rogers. On the dance floor, who is the better dancer? Obviously they are a team, and their actions represent their coordinated movements. It is the same with conflicted couples. Not until one partner sits out the old dance or begins new steps to new music does it become evident that the partner who still moves to the old melody owns the problem. As long as they both engage in maintaining the troubled behavior, they are mutually and equally responsible. Both play the Child's game of "you lose" with the futile hope that "I will win this time."

An important exception to equal responsibility exists when it comes to domestic physical abuse. Although the victim is frequently provocative, such provocation *never* justifies the violence. If the potential perpetrator walks away from the provocation (no longer dancing to the old music), then the "Need-to-be" victim stands out like a sore thumb. Except in the case of physical violence, conflicts are the partners' mutual responsibility, even if one protests that the other one is totally at fault.

Changing for Oneself

It follows that even if one partner makes a 100 percent effort to change, it can count for only 50 percent within the relationship. This does not make the effort valueless; it benefits the growth of the person who makes the effort and contributes to a healthier partnership. Nonetheless, for the relationship ultimately to succeed, the other partner must participate equally. Not unlike volleying in a tennis game, one partner may try to play both sides of the net hoping that somehow such tremendous effort will make a difference and keep the game going. But unless the other person also changes, new solutions are impeded.

When one partner stops playing the game, the interpersonal conflict ceases. The old bumper sticker says, "What If They Gave a War and Nobody Came?" *It takes only one partner to end the conflict, but it takes both partners to improve the relationship.* If conflict is the only glue that holds the relationship together, then resolving the conflict may mean that it will fall apart.

Even if only one person in a relationship makes healthy changes, ultimately those changes will influence the behavior of the other, be it a mate, family member, friend, or coworker. Picture a mobile sculpture—perhaps the huge one by Alexander Calder in the lobby of the National Gallery of Art. The image of the mobile conveys the same power one person can make in a connected system. A resting mobile reflects the exquisite balance between each piece. Such a balance in relationships is best thought of as *homeodynamic* rather than *homeostatic;* the participant(s) preventing change simply expend too much energy to call it static. If any one piece of the mobile's complex assemblage moves, it affects all the other pieces, and a new equilibrium must be found. The structure has changed. The initiator of the change process, if the system accepts the change, creates an intervention from which all may benefit and which none may ignore.

A close-knit immigrant family, unreceptive to any direct outside intervention, may exemplify this notion. If their child comes home from work, school, or therapy with new and helpful ideas, the rest of the family responds because they value their child. On the other hand, if the system does not welcome or allow the change, the person risks becoming a pariah and may be excluded from the group. Even if the system (be it a family, a couple, or a repressive society) exiles the individual, it must expend great energy in reestablishing and maintaining the old, familiar balance to obviate the changed person's influence.

Hillel's Three Questions

By and large, what is ultimately good for one person is likely good for the relationship as well. That is, a partner who operates as an **Adult** and no longer participates in maintaining conflict can encourage and support significant others to find new ways of relating. A self-absorbed, neglectful spouse operates in a self-defeating manner even if he feels content. His mate may accept and even encourage such behavior; but this represents their shared emotional conflict, not their mental health. The long-suffering one who self-sacrifices to accommodate the self-centered other contributes to the relationship's problem. The terms *enabling* or *codependence* describe this process.

Determining what constitutes appropriate behavior in a relationship may be confusing. How can this dilemma of balancing self with others be solved? Is there a guide? I have yet to find a better one than the succinct, triadic inquiries of Hillel, a first century CE rabbi and philosopher:[8]

If I am not for myself, who will be for me?

If I am only for myself, what am I?

If not now, when?

These three short questions powerfully emphasize the importance of self-esteem, avoiding narcissism, and countering procrastination.

When Different Is the Same

The **Child** often plays a trick on the adult to soothe both of them. (I did not capitalize the word *adult* here because I am referring to the aspect of the present self that is controlled by unresolved past conflicts. The use of the capitalized **Adult** is reserved to designate the state of being free of childhood conflicts.) If the adult cannot consciously accept the **Child's** Need cues, the **Child** will allow him to choose the exact opposite—its mirror image. This trick can be illustrated with the following clinical example.

A man who, as a boy, observed his mother denigrate and belittle his father incorporates this image from childhood as the model his **Child** Needs in order to feel at home. Now as an adult he may be resigned to such being his fate. By direct modeling he selects as his mate a woman who, like his mother, Needs to be aggressive while he assumes a subordinate role. This represents a straightforward lock-and-key fit. But if being like his father has become anathema to him, he may say, "I will never allow myself to be treated the way Mother treated Father." Yet this model forms his Need. Instead, he may choose as his wife a subservient woman, not unlike his father, as his wife.

By choosing a woman whose behavior reassures him that he is not the one denigrated because the woman's Child Need dictates that she is, the Child tricks the adult into believing that he is not following the parental model. With this usually unconscious trick of exact oppositeness, sameness is actually established, similar to a mirror reflecting the same but opposite image.

Operating from the unresolved Child's mode of binary/digital thinking, one perceives only two possible choices. In this case the man can behave as his father did, or he can directly reverse the roles if as an adult he recoils from his father's behavior. If the script is not followed, the potential loss of the familiar/familial threatens the Child. "Okay," he may reason, "since the adult me abhors what I Need to have, I will accept his selecting the *exact opposite.*" This is the trick. The use of the mirror image calms the Child while it lulls the adult into thinking that he is nothing like his devalued father.

Many adults unconsciously employ such mirror imaging to be different from an undesired parent-model. For example, a man complains that his wife keeps a messy and disorganized home. Her history reveals that her mother was a meticulous housekeeper, to the point of making their home more like a museum than a living space. She hated her mother's fastidiousness. By keeping a messy home, she makes sure that she is not like her mother. Yet it is her Child's image of mother that precisely dictates how she as an adult maintains her own home. In order to be the exact opposite, the same becomes the guide. This mirroring behavior reflects a complete absence of choice while at the same time seeming to be a radical departure from the familiar. Her Child controls her adult.

Similarly, a wife bitterly bemoans that her husband is a spendthrift and can never keep money in his pocket. The husband describes how his father could make Lincoln on the penny scream with pain from the pinching. The father created the feeling that the family was one small step from the poorhouse. He deprived everyone of everything other than the bare necessities—even though there were, in fact, more than adequate funds. By being a spendthrift, the husband conducts his life *as if* he were nothing like his father. Yet his actions are directly dictated by his father's behavior, only his is the mirror opposite. In this way, the Child compromises his Need for sameness with the adult's wish to be different.

Not only does the exact opposite behavior maintain his father as the model, it also paradoxically threatens to fulfill his childhood's dreaded fear of being broke. As experienced in childhood, in adulthood he maintains home in a way that on the surface seems totally different. But consistent with the paradox of conflict, he has ended up in the exact place he tried to avoid.

In another example, a woman's husband angrily reproaches her for her sloppy mismanagement of the household funds. "If she didn't work at the bank," he grumbles, "we'd be paying a bloody fortune in overdraft fees." Wait a moment. The wife works at a bank? She not only works at a bank, she belongs to the bank's upper echelons and is in charge of handling large sums of money, which she does competently. As a child, she learned from the model of her parent's relationship that a wife was to look good, keep quiet, and stay socially superficial, because wives were expected to have nothing of importance to contribute. Husbands managed anything of importance—particularly money. Therefore as an adult the patient recoiled from such a role. She was determined to be a woman—undeniably capable and substantial—until, that is, she pulls into the driveway of her home. Then a remarkable metamorphosis from the competent adult in the world to the Child at home takes place. Of course, she chose as her husband a man who Needs to see himself as superior. No doubt this reflects the model he internalized from his parents.

When relating from their shared Child Needs, couples are "playing house;" no Adults are present. This is certainly not always the case; instances and circumstances exist when even conflicted couples function well as adults, both together and individually. The shared, unresolved conflicts emanating from childhood emerge under emotionally charged circumstances. It becomes the default setting for their dysfunctional life together as husband and wife.

In a wonderfully succinct four-panel cartoon, Jules Feiffer illustrated the concept of thinking a person can be different by being the exact opposite of the parent he opposes. In the first panel, a woman is shown listing all the undesirable characteristics of her mother. In the subsequent panels, she goes on to say that she therefore raised her daughter, Jennifer, in exactly the opposite way. Each characteristic listed for the daughter is the antithesis of the ones describing her mother. The final panel shows the woman reflecting, "Now my Jennifer is just like my mother."[9]

So why do people in conflict not realize what they are doing? It is because they operate emotionally from their Child self and not from the Adult. From the Child's position at least three crucial factors, discussed earlier, are at play: (1) safety and survival gained through recapitulating the familiar; (2) the use of binary, concrete thought processes; and (3) the perception of having no viable options.

Remember, the Child operates in the binary/digital thought mode of yes/no, all/none, black/white, on/off. Only the Adult has analogue capacity and recognizes that choices exist. Whenever an adult engages in a binary thinking mode, he is in the Child state in which the past predominates over the present. In the Adult state he recognizes that myriad grey tones color the world of human relationships. Very little is ever just black or white, and a spectrum of possible choices exists between extremes.

Occasionally an exception to the powerful influence of past patterning occurs. A young adult leaves home—say, to go to college—mindful of his family's turmoil and conflict. He may say that he does not want his life to be anything like that of his family. During a "honeymoon" period he operates as though he were completely free of the family's conflicts, and he experiences himself as very much the adult. But it is a fragile state. His underlying Needs have been shelved but not resolved. He dates women who are just what he desires in relationships. But because of his unresolved Needs, when it comes to a commitment, lo and behold, all his old patterns re-emerge. He will commit to a woman who has similar unresolved Needs stemming from her own background. The honeymoon is over. They are now *back* in the home they came from—the same home they will make for themselves.

The expression, "It is easy to take the boy out of the family, but it is quite another matter to take the family out of the boy," illustrates this idea. Maya Angelou poignantly demonstrated this in her conversation with Bill Moyer for a 1981 public television program. They were strolling through the small southern town of her childhood, the first time she had been back as an adult. Moyer asked her what it was like to return. She responded with a profound observation: "Do we really ever leave?" Of course, the answer is no, because that early experience remains a part of our total being. The whole gamut of our childhood experiences from the wonderful and pleasant neutral to the *resolved* conflicted memories are incorporated in our **Adult**, while our **Child** represents the unresolved past conflicts' repository. For Angelou, an instance occurred when their stroll took them to the railroad track that had separated the town's blacks from its whites. She could not go further, for in her childhood, it was prohibited for African-Americans to cross the tracks from the "wrong side" without permission. Perhaps the expression "You can never go home again" is best understood as never being able to go back to what we *wish* would have been home. "You can never leave home" more accurately states the permanence of early childhood experiences, dovetailing with what Angelou experienced and observed.

Yesterday's experiences that are desirable and meaningful become incorporated into today's Wants, but those that are unresolved compete for emotional attention in the present. Only with resolution do those Needs become past. The crucial question we must ask ourselves is, "Will I continue to live in the past, or can I risk being in the present and have a new future?"

Splitting the Ambivalence

There are times when a person behaves in a manner contrary to favorable family patterns. A child's rebelling may represent early experimentation with growth, just as some adolescents try different roles that initially may be antithetical to family mores. Take for example a young girl raised in a family with strong positive values regarding personal hygiene, education, honesty, integrity, consideration, ethics, morality, and so forth. Her parents are understandably shocked and confused when one day their daughter brings home a date—a slovenly, ill-kempt, and unemployed guy. Very likely this represents the daughter's attempt to express her own individuality. After all, if she is in lockstep with the family, how can anyone recognize her as a separate person?

Of course the introduction of her primitive friend alarms the parents, who potentially will fall into a trap referred to as *splitting the ambivalence*. There is good and bad in everyone, and therefore mixed feelings abound. It is important for the parents to avoid being the only ones expressing the unpleasant dimension of their feelings about the friend. If they do, the daughter gets away with focusing on just her favorable feelings about him. All the uncomfortable feelings are now in the parent's domain, and the daughter holds only pleasant ones—that is, they have split the ambivalence.

Ideally, the parents would point out that although they may be surprised by the daughter's choice and that her friend is not necessarily the kind of person they would find attractive, no doubt she sees something favorable in him. This way they show respect for her while not agreeing with her choice. Now she has to deal with the unpleasant feelings within herself, since the parents are not going to do it for her, which enables her to say sooner, "He does kind of smell, doesn't he?" rather than, "You just don't understand how wonderful he is."

An elderly woman who lives alone and has two adult children provides another illustration. Her older daughter wants her to go into a retirement home so she can be taken care of and not be a source of worry. The younger daughter respects the mother's competence to assess the situation and make her own decisions. While the first daughter spends many hours bombarding her mother with all the positives of being in a facility, the mother counters, saying that she does not want to give up her privacy, furnishings, or independence. The older daughter's good intentions are lost in the adversarial polarization that takes place.

"I understand my sister wants you to move to a retirement home," the younger daughter says to her mother. "I don't know why you would want to do that."

"Well, I know so many people who are there," the mother counters. "It would be nice to spend time with them. And, you know, I wouldn't have to worry about shopping for food, cooking, or forgetting to take my medications. If I were to fall, someone would be right there to help. They'll let me move in some of my own furniture, just like home, you know." The mother was perfectly aware of all the positives, but they were in the domain of the older, frustrated sister, leaving Mother to focus only on the negatives of moving when talking to the older daughter.

This example can be extrapolated to many other situations. When one partner in a relationship gets caught up in expressing only adverse feelings, it leaves the other partner with just the pleasant ones. What should be an allied relationship becomes adversarial. The adverse consequence of avoiding wrestling with ambivalent feelings is twofold: The problem cannot be resolved, and the potential support from a significant other, now turned adversary, has been lost.

No Negative Feelings

I want to make an important, brief aside. When referring to feelings, I prefer to use terms such as favorable or unfavorable, pleasant or unpleasant, comfortable or uncomfortable, and so on. It is when characterizing views, perceptions, assumptions, or premises that *negative* and *positive* seem appropriate. In ordinary language, we commonly describe unpleasant, painful, or uncomfortable feelings as negative. There is a problem in doing so.

It is not very encouraging or desirable to ask people to experience and express that which is labeled as negative. Considering all feelings, even those generated by negative perceptions, as positive seems preferable, because experiencing and expressing feelings is such an important goal in preventing them from being shunted off as symptomatic behavior. At the very least, we should urge people to avoid the term *negative* when discussing feelings and instead directly call them *painful, unpleasant, uncomfortable*, or whatever the specific feeling being experienced may be.

Life's Laboratory

Marriage affords us the unique opportunity to more fully understand ourselves. This is not always a welcome invitation, because it is precisely our unresolved childhood conflicts that prompted our choice of spouse. Nevertheless, we will never find a better partner in self-discovery than the one who inevitably rings old bells. "He keeps pushing my buttons," a patient may lament, as though it somehow justifies her symptomatic behavior. The button-pushing, bell-ringing metaphor is apt. We have all encountered a doorbell that simply will not ring no matter how often or how vigorously we push the button. If the wiring on the inside no longer connects to the bell, pushing the button on the outside will not make it ring.

In a relationship, it is important for the button-pusher to recognize behavior that may adversely affect his partner and to discontinue such behavior if at all appropriate and possible to do so. However, whether or not the bell sounds has to be the responsibility of the bell's owner, no matter how much button-pushing is going on. Of course, in reality, other people's provocative behavior affects us and may annoy or amuse us, but being annoyed as an **Adult** by others' behavior differs greatly from feeling diminished or devastated by such behavior when one is a child.

I have made up a story, called the "7-Eleven story," which I tell patients to illustrate this concept: A patient arrives a little late for an appointment. Imagine that I respond by telling him that I know that he is late because he stopped on the way to the office and robbed a 7-Eleven store. Reasonably assuming this has absolutely no basis in reality, the patient will respond with a wan smile and look of puzzlement. If I continue my tirade about him being a robber, he might justifiably become annoyed and wonder with what kind of nut he is dealing. At no time will he be distraught, depressed, shamed, or enraged. Why not? My accusation of him being a robber is certainly not benign. The explanation is simply that what comes from the outside—my statement—does *not* resonate with anything within the person. There is no connection. A button has been pushed, but no bell rings.

If whatever comment from another person connects with *unresolved* Child feelings inside, however, the person will react based on his past and once more feel diminished, shamed, hurt, frightened, or helpless. He may defend against those feelings with expressions of anger. "How dare you accuse me of such a thing?" or "You are horrible for what you are saying about me." The still-connected bell rings loudly.

The 7-Eleven story highlights the point that if we resolve old conflicts, then what others say may remind us of the past—of a place we once lived but do not anymore. We may wince at the comments, but we will not collapse in despair, rage, or desperation. So it is not what other people say that determines how we feel or how we respond. It is what we *perceive* the comments to mean, filtered through our past, that rings a bell or not. And if the bell rings, we need to identify what was evoked from our past as if it were still present and not have it determine how we will act. This is the crucial difference between "you hurt me," the statement of the Child, and "I feel hurt," the statement of the Adult.

A child's feelings depend far more on the words and actions of others than do those of a grownup. If you seriously believe that others are totally responsible for making you unhappy, just try asking them, when you are feeling down, to take full responsibility for making you happy. The impotence of their efforts is quickly revealed. Certainly others are relevant to our moods and often contribute greatly one way or another, but they are not in charge.

We can discover the unfinished business of our own growth in the laboratory of our closest relationships. Our mates often evoke intense, unresolved feelings within us. After all, that is why we chose them. At such times, our Child state emerges and we regress to a place in our past. When this happens, our mates may similarly regress, intensifying the conflict. By understanding the process and taking responsibility for our own feelings and behavior, we lessen the intensity and duration of the regression.

Our partners' ability to provide old cues to which we have old responses makes this process of resolution difficult. Our wires are intact and the bell still rings. As I have repeatedly emphasized, we choose our specific partners for this reason: They know exactly which buttons still connect to hot wires, just as we know theirs.

When both partners mutually engage in conflict, the "kids" have pushed the adults aside. Such regression is inevitable and to be expected even as a couple works toward resolving problems. A useful goal is not so much to completely eliminate any regression by either partner but rather to try keeping one **Adult** present at all times. Who this is may vary from time to time and from stress to stress. The inevitable regressions that do occur will then be shorter and less intense.

The Goal of the Adult

In a successful relationship with a shared commitment to the resolution rather than the perpetuation of conflicts, the partners mutually support each other's growth. I have focused on the marital arena, but unresolved issues from the past do not emerge exclusively with our spouses. They can reappear in any significant interactions, such as with parents, friends, bosses, or coworkers—which only emphasizes the importance of taking responsibility for our own feelings and actions.

Past conflicts may be the only thing holding some relationships together. Conflicted Needs act like mortar with bricks. They may bind people, but they also keep them "stuck apart." Resolving conflicts allows for a new way of connecting. This invokes an inherent risk in problem-solving and making changes, since the form of the emerging new relationship cannot be guaranteed. Then again, holding onto conflicts only ensures that the relationship will never improve.

People often ask me if I am a marriage counselor. My reply is that I am a *conjoint therapist*. There is a significant difference. I firmly believe in the importance of maintaining a marriage if at all possible. But my first priority is to help a couple relate to each other in real time, unburdened by undesired past constrictions imposed on the present—that is, relating as one **Adult** to another **Adult**. Once a couple engages in this way, the mortar of conflict dissolves, freeing them to decide what better kind of a bond they wish to develop, if any.

If they choose not to rebond, they can be grateful to each other for mutually helping their relationship transcend old patterns, enabling them to move on to new relationships. In other words, if they have resolved their troubled, shared Needs (driven by desperation) they are now ready to have what they Want (driven by desire) even if it may not be with each other.

Resolving conflicts in one partnership does not guarantee that the next one will be problem-free. Life does not work that way. Even so, problems that Adults face in real time always have the potential for satisfactory resolutions. When two partners engage in mutually respectful negotiation and compromise, they feel valued and allied. In contrast, if problems from the past—the Child—remain unaddressed and unresolved, they tend to be perpetuated in one guise or another with any subsequent partner. The same issues, perhaps clothed in new garb and diluted to some extent from experience and with maturation, nonetheless will keep coming up. The adult's opportunity to become an Adult is then further postponed.

The danger is that *unaddressed* means *unresolved.* And unresolved means *perpetuated.* The new couple may begin to experience the old distress that both thought they had left behind with the divorced "losers." Solving problems by splitting from the previous spouse can create a transient sense of being a "winner"; one imagines that the external change engenders an internal one as well.

I have described a successful relationship process by which both partners join together to resolve their conflicts. What happens if only one partner wants change? Then that person must discontinue his role in the conflicted dance and learn to develop new responses to the powerful, old stimuli coming from his partner. By not taking the old bait, he can keep off the old hooks. Understanding the role each partner played but no longer heeding the call to continue with old patterns means that the past is actually past and no longer interfering with the present. The changed person can now live fully in the present, although unfortunately it may be without the current partner.

We reach a crucial juncture in our psychological growth when our spouses are unwilling or unable to join us in the process. With the recognition that we can be the Adult with Wants and no longer a Child with Needs comes another vital realization: Having no relationship may be better than continuing a bad one. This is the emotional Rubicon we must cross. It means breaking free of the old chains, unintimidated by the zero we must traverse. It answers the question, "How do you win a game called 'you lose'?" Of course, the only way to win is not to play. The Adult's goal is to have successful relationships, free of past conflicts; and if this cannot be reached with the present partner, it may be time to move on.

It Takes so much Work—Is it Worth It?

Couples as well as individuals frequently question whether all the work necessary to solve their problems is really worth the effort. They often think that separating will end their difficulties. For all the reasons described in this chapter, the unresolved conflicts simply get restaged and replayed in subsequent relationships, albeit diluted by whatever general growth the participants have experienced in the meantime. I have come to appreciate that the real requirement for healthy growth is not so much the work to be done with the other person but the work we must do with ourselves. When exposed to the old Need cues proffered by the partner's Child self, a person must exert significant effort to avoid regressing into his own Child part. Collusion keeps the conflict alive. Staying in the here and now as an Adult takes work. *The price of Adulthood is eternal vigilance; you must always know where your Child is.* But the payoff is as invaluable as the rewards of being a grownup.

The Wedding Picture

The following diagram represents a couple's *operational* portrait, their emotional wedding picture, but it also applies to any two people in a significant intimate relationship—regardless of gender. When working with individual patients or with couples, I like to draw this diagram to help clarify and illustrate the mutual mechanisms involved in creating and maintaining their difficulties.

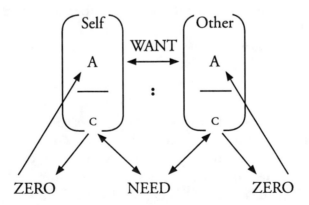

Figure 5-2 The Wedding Picture

An adult's Child seeks a significant other whose Child shares his Need system—*the emotional twinship of couples*—that cues them to "home," or the familiar/familial "safe" place, even if it is constricting, conflicted, painful, and unsatisfying. Abandoning undesired Needs means facing the anxieties of uncertainty—zero—that accompany growth on the path to reach what their Adults mutually Want. Giving up the hope to change the past by repeatedly recreating it and instead accepting what cannot be changed means we are emotionally leaving "home" for the first time— regardless of the age at which this occurs. When the chains that have kept us in our old homes are broken, the feeling is akin to becoming orphaned. To attain what we Want requires our willingness to break free. The path from the Child's Needs to the Adult's Wants goes through zero. Cases are presented in chapter nine to illustrate this.

Masterson, in treating people suffering from disorders of the self, describes how successful therapy helps them experience increasing sadness. Those feelings reach a nadir with the realization that the "tie that binds"[10] us to unresolved Needs must be severed; all the conflicted ways of staying connected must be dissolved. This is a profound step. The tremendous payoff for letting go of the past is the freeing up of emotional resources that can be invested in the present and, thereby, the future.

Some people naturally reach an Adult level of relating because they had a healthy supply of good-enough parenting that allowed for resolution or transformation of their conflicted childhood Needs into what they Want as adults. Those not so fortunate must grieve the loss of the old and abandon any hope of having a different past—going through some form of zero—to reach Adulthood. The game of trying to create a new past is, by definition, a losing proposition, no matter how it is played.

Courage to Change

When we are unhappy with our circumstances, we often speak enthusiastically of the importance of change. Realizing that this entails giving up unresolved Needs, we try to have change on the one hand without doing anything different on the other. Therein lies the essence of conflict in the process of change: The Adult (Wanting change) runs into the tenacity of the Child (Needing nothing to be different). The tension between these two states generates both the motivation for and the resistance to growth.

Emotional growth unquestionably requires courage. Think of how incredibly brave were medieval sailors imbued with the idea of Cosmas Indicopleustes that the earth is flat—yet they were willing to risk sailing beyond the horizon into the abyss.[11] I therefore liken change to falling off the edge of a cliff (as referred to in chapter four). It does not take a long time. But our attempt to keep the land of the past in sight impedes our voyage in the present. The courage to grow includes both getting to and through zero by breaking free of old bonds and continuing to move in increasingly positive ways, even when we lose sight of "home port."

In a recent television program about the animated 3-D film *Coraline* its writer and director, Henry Selick, said that when he was young, he thought bravery meant doing things without having any fear. Now as an adult he realizes that bravery is all about being afraid but going ahead and doing what has to be done anyway. If all of us who want to change and anxiously stare at the void—the zero we have to traverse—remember that bravery means going ahead and doing what we have to do in spite of our fear, we can embrace our anxiety knowing that without fear there is no challenge, and without challenge there is no change.

Salvador Minuchin, a pioneer in the field of family therapy, in a presentation to a group of therapists offhandedly commented that he had been married to seven women. The audience gasped. He quickly added that perhaps he should explain. In his multiple decades of marriage, he could recognize the stages of growth his wife had gone through and the metamorphoses she had undergone: from the young bride, to a young wife, to a mother, and so forth. He felt most fortunate to have been able to grow with her, he said, otherwise they could have found themselves growing apart. Though such an outcome would have been sad and unfortunate, the consolation would have been the emphasis they put on *growing*, not on *apart*.[12] Now that takes courage.

Patterns of Relating

Below I have characterized relationships with a number of configurations, using a simple line to represent each person. These schematics are particularly applicable in describing marital relationships, but we can recognize them in other social contexts as well.

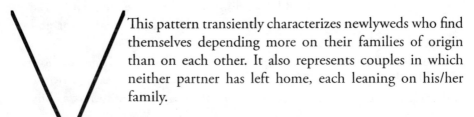

This pattern transiently characterizes newlyweds who find themselves depending more on their families of origin than on each other. It also represents couples in which neither partner has left home, each leaning on his/her family.

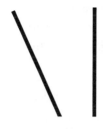

Here one partner (left) is dependent on others. This is tolerated, even fostered, by the one who seems independent (right). The leaning partner bears the onus of *immature dependency* or weakness.

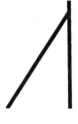

This is similar to the above. The leaning partner seems dependent on the one standing. This pattern may conceal the reality that the leaner could in fact be the one whose strength is used to hold up the one seeming to be the strong one.

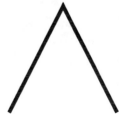

Here both are totally dependent on each other. The dependence is mutual and immature, inhibiting either partner from growing.

In this pattern, both partners seem to be standing on their own two feet. But their postures represent mutual *independence* and demand a safe distance be maintained at all times.

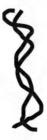

This configuration is the antithesis of the one above. Instead of fearing closeness, both partners must cling to each other to feel whole, often becoming completely enmeshed without any individual selves.

This is the optimum pattern of two people who can stand on their own *and* be intimate, representing a state of personal *autonomy* and shared *mature dependence*

Figures 5-3 Patterns of Relating

These simple diagrams enable couples to recognize the shape of their own relationship patterns and have an image of an optimum goal for which to strive.

The Need system and its associated patterns of relating get passed on uninterrupted from one generation to the next, either directly or in the mirror opposite fashion described previously. A young woman growing up in the Appalachian Mountains vividly illustrated this when relating her family history. She reported that in her culture, females normally marry around twelve years of age and begin having children at thirteen. Because of this, she had direct knowledge of her family's relationship patterns going back seven generations—five of which she actually knew and had observed. Her description reflected the way the conflict pendulum simply oscillates from one generation to the next, with the same distress theme being passed on from mother to daughter and father to son—or the reverse, from mother to son and father to daughter.

When couples recognize that their families' patterns of relating have likely been passed on from generation to generation, they gain a greater, fault-free appreciation for just how tenaciously these patterns have been adhered to and repeated. They may then determine that they will not be yet another generation visiting unresolved conflicts, no matter how honestly arrived at, on their children.

Memetics

The transmitting of "existence" models or behavior patterns from parents to their children may be conceptualized as a type of psychological genetics. These patterns can become as emotionally entrenched as genetics are entrenched biologically. The perpetuation of troubled patterns ceases only when and if someone says, "The buck stops here. I will not allow my kids to endure the unresolved problems I have inherited from my parents." This concept of generational transmission has been advanced in the fast-growing but little-known field called *memetics*.

Richard Dawkins coined the word memetics to signify the science of memes, derived from the word *memory*. Dawkins used memetics to refer to "ideas, habits, and beliefs that are passed on from person to person by imitation. Ideas, styles, and beliefs pass from person to person and from generation to generation. What genes are to our bodies, memes are to human culture and mind. Beliefs that survive are not necessarily true, rules that survive are not necessarily fair, and rituals that survive are not necessarily necessary."[13]

Dawkins's observation does not emphasize Needs—the imperative of perpetuating underlying emotional conflicts. My focus has been on our need to maintain continuity with the past in order to survive—even if this ends up killing us. The continuing use of warfare to resolve conflicts and ideological culture clashes resulting from rigid fundamentalism are macro-examples of this process. At any level of society from individuals to nations, whenever feelings of uncertainty and fears of the unknown prohibit change and stop the act of questioning and exploring, the process of blind perpetuation is in play.

How can we change? How do we succeed in casting off constraints that have been carried forward from an earlier time in life? How do we come to appreciate that the excitement of growth offsets the fear of change? Through life experiences, we may spontaneously recognize that old perceptions and behaviors artificially limit our choices. While there are many roads to Rome, I focus specifically in the next two chapters on the enterprise of the various psychotherapies.

CHAPTER SIX

An Overview of Psychotherapy

As I introduce a general overview of psychotherapy in this and the following chapter, I want to emphasize that psychotherapy, with all its various techniques, has a primary goal: to help us make the transition from perpetuating a conflicted past to achieving a fulfilling present; to break the "secure" chains of childhood conflicts; to go through zero; and to gain the freedom to pursue what we Want.

In the *History of Psychiatry,* Alexander and Seleznick quote this excerpt from Aristophanes' *The Clouds,* in which Socrates tries to solicit from Strepsiades just what his concerns might be:

Soc: Come, lie down here.

Strep: What for?

Soc: Ponder awhile over matters that interest you.

Strep: Oh, I pray not there.

Soc: Come, on the couch!

Strep: What a cruel fate.

Soc: Ponder and examine closely, gather your thoughts together, let your mind turn to every side of things. If you meet with difficulty, spring quickly to some other idea; keep away from sleep.

In this remarkable dialogue so reminiscent of the psychoanalyst-patient interaction, Strepsiades thinks of stopping the movement of the moon. When asked why he would wish to do so, he replies that with the cessation of the moon's movement, there would be no months, and his monthly bills would never come due.[1] Clearly some things never change.

As social beings, we have a natural desire to seek solace from one another, especially when feeling troubled. The previous dialogue and the following examples illustrate this very human characteristic. When feeling distressed, at some point all of us have sought guidance, comfort, or reassurance from someone else; most of us have also been similarly approached. An old *New Yorker* cartoon showed a man seated at a bar. The bartender, towel in hand wiping a glass, says, "Sorry Mac, the guy who handles marital issues is out today. I only deal with existential distress." It is not unusual to hear that someone boarded a bus, sat down next to a receptive-looking person, related the most intimate details of his troubles, and then got off the bus feeling much better. Though such encounters may have a therapeutic quality, and certainly benefits can ensue from them, they do not constitute the specific phenomenon of psychotherapy.

Psychotherapy—A Unique Triad

Using Martin Buber's terms[2] and Ralph Greenson's ideas,[3] I delineate in the following diagram the aspects of the special relationship that uniquely distinguish the enterprise called psychotherapy:

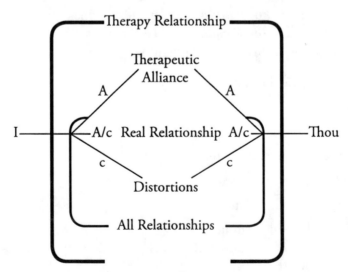

Figure 6-1 Psychotherapy Triad

All human interactions consist of two levels of simultaneous experience. One is the here-and-now interaction that constitutes the *real relationship,* and the other is the *distorted (transferential) relationship.* In the real relationship, both parties recognize each other as adults, appreciating the Adult and the Child aspects each brings to the interaction but continually trying to relate to each other as Adults. The more they interact on the Adult level, the more endearing, valuable, and meaningful the relationship becomes and the longer it can last. This is the stuff of solid friendships. Paradoxically, in psychotherapy, unlike in any other relationship, the sooner this qualitative level is reached, the sooner the relationship ends.

The second, distorted level of everyday social intercourse consists of interactions in the present that are filtered internally through the lens of past experiences. These then-and-there perceptions color the here-and-now to varying degrees—very little in some cases, completely in others. The extent of the coloration depends on the level of each person's unresolved conflict as well as the stress generated in the interaction. In therapy, this distortion is commonly referred to as *transference,* the distortion the patient(s) bring(s) to the interaction, and *countertransference,* the distortion originating from within the therapist. Although these constructs refer to evoked feelings, it is not the feelings that are of concern in therapy but rather the behaviors that may be enacted because of these feelings.

Distinguishing psychotherapy from any other relationship requires the unique addition of a third level to the ordinary two-level interaction I just described. Therapy *must* contain this third level: the *therapeutic alliance.* By virtue of specific training and licensure, society designates a person as a healer/consultant/therapist and those who seek assistance as the patients/clients/consultees. The patient comes to the therapist for help with thoughts, feelings, and/or behaviors that cause or contribute to difficulties in some sphere of the patient's life. These difficulties may be personal, social, familial, and/or occupational. Legal requirements, ethical constraints and standards, and the therapist's theoretical orientation govern the therapeutic alliance. Both parties consent to the therapeutic engagement, its rules, goals, and limitations, which necessitates a modicum of the patient's Adult. "I know I must have help, and I'll accept it from you, the therapist."

If, by his actions, the therapist breaches legal and ethical standards, he ruptures the therapeutic alliance, and therapy ceases. Similarly, a patient engaging in unlawful or egregiously disruptive behavior may bring therapy to an end. A natural corollary follows this discussion: The therapeutic alliance designates the patient as a full partner in the therapeutic process. Nonetheless the therapist must always retain his professional integrity even though the patient may vacillate between manifestations of his Child self and his emerging Adult being. The patient's welfare should remain the focus of the entire enterprise. Berne succinctly and humorously said, "If the therapist uses the patient for his own therapy, he should be prepared to pay the patient his usual fee!"[4]

The Necessity of Theory

In order to establish and maintain a therapeutic alliance, the therapist must have a coherent frame of reference or a theory with which he can formulate an understanding of what may be causing the patient's problem. The theory dictates and guides the necessary treatment considerations and supports the therapist's belief that he can be helpful to his patient.

There is a curious truth about theories: They do not ultimately have to be true. Rather a theory provides the practitioner with a structure by which he can organize his interactions, understanding, and treatment of the patient, as well as a *conviction* that he will help the patient alleviate his suffering.

Bloodletting illustrates the idea that a theory does not conclusively have to be proven true or even beneficial. At one time in medicine, this was the treatment of choice for a wide variety of problems. Only retrospectively do we know that more people may have been harmed than cured by bloodletting. Radical surgeries for cancer and lobotomies for severe psychiatric disorders which only worsened the patients' condition or quality of life exemplify contemporary but now abandoned medical interventions. One of the oldest known surgical procedures, trephening, involves cutting a hole in the person's skull to release "offending spirits." Five-thousand-year-old skulls have been found with clear evidence of such treatments. We now know that the high-fat, dairy diets once recommended to ulcer patients increase stomach acid as well as elevate bad cholesterol levels. No one knew then that ulcers result from a bacterial infection. At the time, practitioners absolutely believed these treatments were *de rigueur*. Now the modalities may seem irrational, bizarre, or even barbaric, but they permitted the doctor to approach the patient genuinely convinced that his treatment would, if not heal the patient, then at least relieve his suffering.

Psychotherapy has also evolved over time. For example, in the early nineteenth century, psychotic individuals were placed in chairs and spun to the point of dizziness—even vomiting—and thereby treated, if not cured. Patients thus treated may well have learned quickly to suppress any expression of symptoms, lest they be "treated" again. Nonetheless, therapists of the time earnestly believed, based on their theories, that they benefited their patients. Psychoanalysis for the treatment of severe obsessive-compulsive disorder was discontinued because a better understanding of the condition's physiology evolved, along with more effective behavioral treatments and medications. Similarly, homosexuality, once thought to be a pathological state, is now recognized (except by a few retrogressive therapists and social and religious institutions) as a normal developmental variation. Freud made this point eloquently when he wrote to the American mother of a homosexual son and explained that the young man did not have a disorder requiring treatment.[5] The rest of psychiatry took a few decades to catch up.

For a therapist to be effective, he must have a theory. At the same time, he should be prepared to abandon that theory if a better one becomes available. This requires of the therapist the same kind of courage to change that is asked of the patient. After all, therapists are human, just like patients, and we all struggle in letting go of thoughts, feelings, and behavior that have guided and informed us but no longer prove useful or effective. Transitioning from the past security of now-obsolete beliefs involves—for patient and therapist alike—the willingness to go through zero to achieve something more positive and effective. Usually we first incorporate such transitions intellectually; emotional understanding comes later.

Accepting Loss

The natural rhythms of life between the constants of birth and death involve change, the third constant. In the face of change, our ability to adapt determines how we emotionally approach life's seasons and new situations. One part of us tries to keep change at bay, which can lead to conflict if we no longer desire what we attempt to preserve. Then avoiding the dreaded feelings of hopelessness and helplessness dictate our actions. Another part of us accepts the inevitability of change; we adapt and mold what we value and allow those values to find meaningful expression in the new circumstance.

When unresolved Needs constrain the person because letting go would mean having to accept loss, he may re-create past scenarios in the present with the hope that "this time I will prevail." Therapy enables the patient's **Adult** to observe, understand, and modify or discontinue this recapitulation. The person can then move on in life, able to tolerate the loss that accompanies growth. Similar intense feelings may be generated by both experiences, but there is a world of difference between a *breakdown* (being controlled by the past) and a *breakthrough* (taking charge of the past). The latter involves giving up painful, self-defeating ways of relating and troubled sets of relationships for more appropriate ones as we progress in our lives.

The essence of Hinduism, expressed in the *Bhagavad Gita* and succinctly condensed here, is "attach, detach, transcend." We cannot survive if we do not attach, and we cannot grow (transcend) if we do not detach. Judith Viorst expressed the importance of tolerating feelings of detachment in her well-titled book *Necessary Losses*.[6] Ramen's expression "there is no healing without grieving"[7] also emphasizes the importance of tolerating the sadness of loss. If tears are shed, they are tears of resolution, not resignation.

We often confuse such sadness with depression, but there is a distinct difference between the two. When we are sad, we retain the belief that whatever we changed or gave up—voluntarily or inevitably—will somehow improve our lives. *Our hope survives our loss.* On the other hand, when depression overcomes us in the face of loss, we abandon hope. Take, for example, the child who has grown, matured, and is now going off to college. Though the parents and adult child may feel loss and sadness, they also appreciate the appropriateness of those feelings. In a healthy relationship, neither parent nor child would do anything to interfere with these natural feelings. Conversely, if the parents fear that their child's growth will leave them bereft of purpose and value, they may attempt to block his leaving or become despairing and depressed. There is a time for all things, it says in Ecclesiastes 3:1, including a time for attaching, a time for detaching, and a time for transcending. Grief and sadness reasonably accompany any loss without ever becoming depression. The equations below distinguish between these two states:

Sadness - Hope = Depression

Depression + Hope = Sadness

Four Essential Components

All therapies, when competently and ethically conducted, utilize four essential components in varying degrees depending on the particular therapy: *confrontation, exploration, separation,* and *application.*

Confrontation refers to stating the patient's problem in as forthrightly a fashion as possible. It does not imply, nor is it intended to mean, a confrontation in any political or adversarial sense. Obviously an unstated problem cannot be resolved. All therapies have in common the need to elucidate the difficulty for which the patient solicits help. Confrontation means facing the very issues that prompted the patient to seek therapy.

Exploration involves a discussion of how the problem developed in the first place and how it now manifests itself. This step may be very brief, as in the behavior modification modalities and some other forms of therapy that do not delve into the historical and developmental aspects of the patient's life. It can also be very extensive, as in psychoanalysis, in which exploration forms the bulk of the work.

Separation means the various ways the therapist attempts to delineate the patient's past from his present by distinguishing the Child's feelings and behaviors from the Adult's—demarcating the then and there from the here and now. All therapies aspire to achieve this distinction, although methods vary widely.

Application means the patient applies what he has learned in therapy in his everyday life. It is an essential component of successful therapy. Some therapists may hold that whatever the patient does outside the session is of no concern to the therapist. I hope this is an antiquated notion. If the therapist has no concern about the patient's application in life of what he has worked on in his sessions, then what the therapist practices is not therapy. If the therapist engages in only the first three steps in whatever appropriate proportions but neglects to focus on application, then the patient gains an important educational experience at best. At worst, the experience is vitiated.

Psychoanalysis

Often a great deal of confusion and occasionally derision accompanies the study of psychoanalysis. But psychoanalysis has a far greater meaning, influence, and applicability than is usually ascribed to it and can be broadly divided into four separate, important areas: *treatment, theory, teaching, and research.*

First, psychoanalysis has come under evaluative scrutiny as a means of treatment, and many questions have been raised about its efficacy. The considerable amount of time required—three to four sessions a week for a number of years—along with the associated expense make psychoanalysis generally less available even for patients who may be considered good candidates for the treatment.

Second, psychoanalysis represents a viable and important theoretical basis for understanding the development of personalities and psychopathology—particularly as it has evolved and incorporated contributions and discoveries from many other disciplines.

Third, psychoanalysis is an experiential teaching modality. Therapists in training often undergo analysis to learn psychoanalytic techniques experientially. In the process, one hopes as patients they will resolve any personal conflicts that might interfere with their professional practices. Similarly, some medical educators have suggested that every medical student should have to be a patient before being allowed to graduate to gain a real understanding of what it means to lie in a hospital bed and be dependent on others for care. Physicians who have themselves been hospitalized acknowledge greater awareness and empathy as a result of their experiences as patients. The psychotherapist's general sensitivity is likewise enhanced through his own therapy experience.

Fourth, psychoanalysis is a valuable and often unappreciated research tool. Poorly understood conditions can be extensively explored for their psychological components with this technique. Robert Stoller's studies of transsexuals as well as his work on the development of gender identity are outstanding examples.[8]

We may better appreciate the rich contributions of psychoanalysis if we keep in mind all four arenas in which it has been fruitfully employed.

The Eclectic Loop

In this section I bring the individual back into central focus and place all the therapies in the context of the patient and his problems.

Human behavior is neither random nor capricious. Our behavior tells as rich a story as do our words. Moreover, our behavioral story, often coded and sometimes misunderstood, contains what we find most significant, though it is often excluded from our verbal communication.

How our perceptions and feelings influence our behavior is shown by what I call the *eclectic loop* (pictured below). It starts with a person's perceptions. The perceptions generate feelings, which drive behavior. We perceive, we feel, and we act. All actions have some kind of outcome. These results reinforce the underlying motivating perceptions, feelings, and behaviors. The reinforcing cycle connecting these four elements constitutes the eclectic loop.

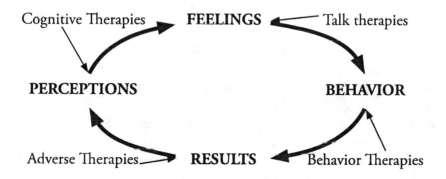

Figure 6-2 The Eclectic Loop

All therapies have a common goal of *breaking the loop* when the established cycle creates and maintains symptoms. In the broadest terms, all therapies can be divided into four major groups: cognitive, talk, behavioral, and aversive, shown above at the point where they act in breaking the loop. Each of these will be addressed following the discussion of how the loop functions.

A very simple example will serve to illustrate the loop's workings (depicted with dark lines). A student perceives himself to be capable and competent at mathematics. This favorable perception leads to his feeling confident and at ease with an upcoming exam. He expresses his confidence behaviorally by preparing for the test: studying and reviewing the material and doing the practice problems. As a result, he receives a good grade on the test. The original perception of competence is thereby reinforced, exemplifying the positive functioning of the loop, the reinforcement of favorable perceptions.

Take the contrary starting perception. A student perceives himself as incompetent in math and may suppress or repress these uncomfortable feelings. Whenever feelings are pushed down, undesirable behavior rises up as the expression of those feelings. The hydraulic model, referred to in Chapter Four, showed how unacknowledged feelings simply transform into behavior (acting out) or bodily symptoms (somatization). Because of his general discomfort with the subject, this student dismisses the importance of studying and may rationalize that relaxing the mind better prepares him for the exam. Perhaps going to a movie instead of studying would be a good idea, he reasons. As a result, he fails the exam. His original perception of incompetence is thereby reinforced.

Earlier I stressed how our unresolved conflicts, through *suppression, repression,* or *sublimation* of feelings, commandeer our behavior. Through sublimation, we channel conflict into constructive outlets that may allow us to function successfully in society without ever addressing the underlying issues. For example, an artist, abused as a child by his mother, uses his canvases as an outlet for feelings of rage, pain, turmoil, and helplessness associated with those experiences. The public clamors for his work, which commands significant prices. Thus his conflict has a societal outlet that is applauded and valued. The favorable feedback seemingly overwhelms the negative perceptions that he has sublimated.

For some, this may be resolution enough for the emotional conflicts. Alas, it is not enough for this artist. Fears of being close to a warm and giving woman dominate his private life. In relationships with healthy women, he feels strange, awkward, and apprehensive. Although an intimate, loving relationship is what he Wants, his Need for abuse becomes manifest in choosing women who are cold, punishing, and withholding. The behavior expresses his Child's expectations and perceptions of a relationship with a significant woman (mother). As a consequence, he feels as unloved as he had been as a child. He continually reinforces his worst expectations. The only difference now is that he feels in charge and can leave the relationship as soon as it becomes unbearable. His behavior demonstrates a sublimated resolution of his childhood experiences in his profession but a perpetuation of the conflict in his personal life.

A core truth emerges from understanding the way the eclectic loop works: *Conflict always paints us into the very corner we are trying to avoid.* As illustrated in the foregoing examples, we operate, knowingly or not, with self-fulfilling prophecies—good or bad. Conflicts not dealt with affect our perceptions and start the cascade that paradoxically results in reinforcing the conflicts. If where the person is in his life contrasts with where he says he would like to be, we have to wonder why. What Needs keep him where he is and prevent him from going where he Wants to be? The answer lies in understanding which perceptions and feelings drive the behavior that produces results antithetical to his desires—that is, the eclectic loop.

Dynamic Formulation

The *dynamic formulation*[9] is a straightforward hypothesis that attempts to describe the central theme motivating the patient's behavior and his resultant problems. The therapist derives the formulation from the information obtained about the patient, which comes from three sources: The therapist's exploration of the patient's history, his observations of the patient in the consultation room, and his emotional experience while being with the patient. All three sources provide behavioral information in addition to the verbal content of the history. (On some occasions, other parties—spouses, relatives, friends, and authorities—provide a fourth source of input.) In taking the patient's history, the therapist actually accumulates a whole series of behavior-resultant paradigms. What did the person do, when did he do it, what was it like emotionally (for the patient directly and for the therapist while listening), and what were the consequences of what was done? Then, going back to the eclectic loop, the therapist can theorize about the nature of the patient's perceptions and feelings that are being reinforced by his behaviors and their results.

An analogy might be useful to further illustrate that much of the important data a therapist collects are nonverbal. If we watch a person on TV with the sound turned off, we must pay special attention to what he does—his behavior, demeanor, facial expressions, and so on—to fully understand what is being communicated. Similarly, the therapist must keenly attend to the patient's behavior—his body language—as well as verbal content and tone. In doing so, the therapist tries to understand the what and why of the patient's behavior, especially if it contradicts the patient's stated desires. By looking at the corner into which the patient has figuratively painted himself, the therapist can discern the underlying conflict. When he has formulated his theory, this statement of what makes the person function symptomatically becomes the dynamic formulation.

A good formulation is expressed in ordinary language, free of jargon and technical terms and simple enough for any reasonably intelligent adolescent to understand. It need not be more than a sentence or two in length; and it should be a clear enunciation of the therapist's understanding of what drives the patient's problems. When spoken in plain language and shared with the patient, the dynamic formulation helps the patient draw on his healthy Adult to better join in the therapy process. The therapist may say, "Here is what seems to be your problem." This is shared as a speculation, hunch, or hypothesis derived from the patient's history and distilled through the therapist's clinical experience. The therapist should never pontificate. His dynamic formulation may not ultimately be correct, but it forms a starting point for the shared venture. It also helps the therapist in deciding what kinds of interventions may be most useful.

For example, a patient reports feeling despondent about his relationship with women. He says he felt similarly fifteen years earlier when a woman he had dated rejected him. Two years ago he met a woman whom he believed would become his wife. They continued dating and spoke of marriage. He was very happy—until his brother started to take an interest in the same woman, began to date her, and subsequently married her. Each time the patient saw the two together, he had to face his lost dreams. He suffered silently, without ever saying anything to either of them or anyone else. He came to therapy because he felt acute pain after learning that they were expecting a child—the child that should have been his. The patient's brother had always been treated as the special one. The parents berated the patient for never being as intelligent, good-looking, or capable as his brother. The therapist's dynamic formulation hypothesized that a part of the patient (the Child) perceived himself as the family did—that he was not good enough to deserve having what he desired.

I use this example to illustrate the straightforward statement that reflects an understanding of what the patient perceives about himself and expresses through his behavior, both socially and occupationally. The value of the dynamic formulation is in its attempt to answer the question, "What accounts for the symptomatic behavior observed?" It should also help to guide the therapist's interactions with and treatments of the patient. For example, this patient did not keep his second appointment. Given the specific hypothesis used to understand him—his not being good enough to have what he wants—the therapist took the initiative and called him. Patient and therapist were subsequently able to discuss the missed appointment as representing a powerful nonverbal communication. Did the therapist care if he showed up? Did the therapist also believe that the patient had no worth, as he thought everyone else did in his life?

Given a different patient and a different dynamic formulation or hypothesis, it might have been totally inappropriate to call about the missed appointment. But in this case, the understanding of the patient reflected in the formulation dictated the importance of letting the patient know the therapist's concern.

Sometimes simply doing no harm is the only possible avenue for the therapist, yet it potentially becomes the beginning of the help that may follow. This patient who struggles with the feeling of never being good enough has experienced a therapist who affirmed his worthiness by calling him. The patient's action, missing the appointment, has now had a totally different result than he ever anticipated. At the very least, the therapist has avoided becoming yet another rejecter in the patient's life. The seeds of awareness that things could perhaps be different for the patient have been planted and may take root at some future time.

Synthesizing a dynamic formulation is vital *regardless of the mode of therapy employed.* Even so, some therapists do not develop such a formulation and may possibly proceed without one; they might simply offer what they believe to be generally helpful. This constitutes a one-size-fits-all approach that can, in fact, help some people some of the time. However, with a formulation, the therapist can integrate his own understanding of the patient and utilize the mode of therapy that will most likely be helpful, and then fine-tune it to fit that particular patient's problem. If nothing else—as illustrated in the foregoing example—the dynamic formulation helps the therapist to avoid falling into the trap of simply continuing in therapy the same negating experiences the patient has had in all his other relationships.

The four major therapy categories I noted earlier, corresponding to the diagram of the eclectic loop, are discussed in the next section. All therapies attempt to break a patient's symptomatic cycle, but at different points in the eclectic loop. Sharing an understanding of the loop's function with the patient may facilitate the therapeutic alliance and foster the patient's participation in the therapy enterprise. At the very least, understanding the way the loop works can help a therapist avoid inadvertently reinforcing the very problem the patient experiences. If the therapist cannot be of help, then at least he should do no harm.

Breaking the Eclectic Loop

Understanding the nature of the patient's problem—the dynamic formulation—guides the therapist in making interventions that are most likely to be helpful. Here I return to discussing the various categories of therapies that may be employed in attempting to disrupt the symptomatic, reinforcing loop. Therapy helps the patient develop new perceptions, feelings, and behavior and provides an opportunity for him to change negative cycles to positive ones. The many types of therapy fit at one point or another in the eclectic loop; each employs its own individual methodology to break the symptomatic repetition.

Cognitive behavioral techniques focus on the negative perceptions that give rise to regressive feelings. By changing those adverse assumptions, the patient will feel differently, and those feelings in turn prompt changes in his behavior. It is useful to consider the possibility that *feelings may be perfectly reasonable responses to perfectly unreasonable assumptions.* If a patient perceives that "I can never be loved," a sense of resignation and despair naturally follows from this false premise. Because such thoughts or perceptions were once learned and experienced as real in childhood, and invested with the power that comes from learning under the unique circumstances of idealized optionlessness, they become incredibly powerful and difficult to change.

Cognitive behavior therapy uses what has been called the three C's: *catch, challenge, and change.* Catch the negative thought, then challenge that thought using all the positive truths that exist, thereby countering the premise; change naturally follows. Unchallenged, a corrosive thought will naturally lead to corrosive feelings. Behavior motivated by those feelings leads to unattractive results. Those results reinforce the initial negative perception—and the not-so-merry merry-go-round makes yet another full turn. This is but one example of a number of protocols with which cognitive behavioral therapists approach different clinical problems.[10]

When the patient learns to recognize faulty perceptions and how to use techniques to counter those perceptions, his feelings will be modified and his behavior adjusted, and the results will no longer create the illusion that the original faulty perceptions had validity. In this way, the eclectic loop changes from continually reinforcing the very problems causing the patient's suffering.

Talk therapy, another possible intervention in the loop, focuses on verbalizing feelings rather than having them expressed through behavior. When people think of therapy, they usually think of talk therapy. The stereotype of the psychotherapies, it is probably the most common as well as the oldest form of therapy, as the dialogue between Socrates and Strepsiades at the beginning of this chapter illustrates. Freud was convinced that there is something crucial, both biologically and psychologically, about verbalizing conflicts and thereby reducing their intensity. Being able to put our feelings into words creates a sense of mastery and contributes to the development of a cohesive narrative so that we can make sense of our lives. Recall that Adam's first task was to name all the animals. By putting names to things, we begin to create a sense of control over the threatening unknown.

Experiencing and expressing emotions verbally becomes an antidote to destructive behaviors. What does not get *talked* out gets *acted* out. Freud described this phenomenon and its manifestations in the patient's life as well as in the consultation room relationship.[11] Patients often say that they cannot remember certain aspects of their childhoods. By observing the patient's behavior, however, the therapist can identify the uncomfortable feelings not remembered, because the patient acts them out.[12] This is the rationale underlying the Gestalt therapy of Fritz Perls. According to Perls, no history-taking is necessary, only close observation of the patient's present behaviors with the therapist. The conflicts are clearly in motion. With the therapist's help, the patient can verbalize the behaviorally associated emotions, gain awareness of his problems, and thereby have the opportunity to change.[13]

No therapist, whatever his theoretical approach, is interested in the patient's past in general. As stated earlier, it is only the patient's unresolved past conflicts that are the focus of therapy, because they interfere with his present functioning. Unwanted significant feelings cannot simply be dismissed from awareness except by (conscious or subconscious) suppression or (unconscious) repression. With either course, the conflicted feelings become expressed through behavior. The therapeutic goal is to encourage the verbal expression and understanding of feelings in order to free the patient from communicating them with emotionally commandeered behavior. Now able to talk out and no longer having to act out conflicts, the patient is freed to express a panoply of favorable perceptions and feelings. This begins the reinforcing, restorative (analeptic) cycle.

As a corollary to cognitive behavioral therapy with its focus on perceptions leading to feelings, the verbalizing of feelings allows one to become aware of underlying perceptions. The patient may ask himself, "On what assumptions am I basing my feelings?" Although feelings are always valid, the past perceptions forming them may no longer be true. A person who states, "I feel helpless, but I know that in fact I am not," understands this concept.

Behavior-modifying therapies endeavor to create new results from changes in behavior, thereby breaking the loop at this junction. Engaging in favorable, new behaviors results in more pleasing outcomes. Thus underlying perceptions and feelings are countered by new, positively reinforcing results derived from the new behaviors. For example, a group of depressed individuals were asked to simply smile when encountering others, which was the antithesis of what they felt like doing. Once they did this consistently they began to feel less depressed because of the nature of the reactions of others; a smile led to a smiling response. That in turn led to a change in the underlying sense of self, countering the depression-producing perceptions.[14] Put more simply, emotion follows motion. As Alcoholics Anonymous says, "Fake it till you make it."

In every form of competent therapy, the therapist responds in a manner different from what one would expect in any other relationship. For instance, a patient comes into the office swearing at the therapist. The therapist replies, "Something must be upsetting you. Let's discuss it." This contrasts with the previously experienced negative reaction, which has become the expected one. Recall the man who missed his next appointment and received a call from the therapist rather than being ignored, as he expected. The therapist's statement reflects acceptance, the willingness to listen, and the attempt to understand the patient, all of which contribute to disrupting the patient's otherwise negatively reinforcing loop. Those adept in behavior modification techniques use a wide variety of similar approaches to various problematic behaviors.

Aversive techniques attempt to disrupt any pleasurable results produced by undesirable behavior. Antabuse, for example, produces a noxious physiologic state in a person who ingests alcohol after taking it. This method, no longer widely used, helps alcoholics avoid drinking. The toxicity anticipated or actually experienced replaces whatever pleasurable feelings the alcohol produces. Similarly, individuals who take pleasure in such inappropriate behavior as viewing naked children for prurient reasons have been treated with electric shock while viewing such pictures. The pain produced by the shock replaces previously pleasurable feelings.

The eclectic loop, a powerful tool in maintaining and reinforcing favorable perceptions, must be broken when the cycle reinforces pain and distress. This often requires professional assistance. By breaking the loop between perceptions and feelings, the therapist helps the patient examine, challenge, and change perceptions, which leads to new feelings, behavior, and results. When feelings and their perceptions are expressed verbally in talk therapy, different behaviors ensue with new, desired results. With behavior modification, new behaviors produce new results, which no longer slavishly express symptoms. When results no longer propagate troubled perceptions, feelings, and behaviors, new outcomes follow: Painful feelings for those who watch child pornography and those who drink alcohol while on Antabuse. All therapies, each focusing on one of the four components of the loop, act to help a person break past chains and develop a healthy cycle of favorable perceptions, gratifying feelings, enhancing behaviors, and fulfilling results.

Regardless of the particular mode of therapy employed, the therapist always attempts to respond to the patient in a helpful way. However, an important caveat is that reasonable limitations and certain exceptions apply. If a patient engages in destructive behavior, for example, the therapist, not unlike anyone else, must act to protect himself, his property, and the patient from the destructiveness. Once safety is reestablished, the therapist and the patient can begin to examine the meaning of the behavior.

I will focus in the next chapter on specific ideas, techniques, and adjuncts to therapy that I have found useful in understanding the therapeutic process. These are all oriented toward breaking old chains, going through zero, and having what is Wanted.

CHAPTER SEVEN

Selected Psychotherapy Topics

In this chapter I present some specific impressions and concepts of otherwise common ideas as well as some entirely new formulations regarding the psychotherapy endeavor. I emphasize that the ultimate goal of therapy is to help people make the difficult emotional journey of letting go of the old Need bonds, going through the zero of uncertainty, and having support on their way to reaching what they Want.

Ultra-Brief Therapy

The topic of ultra-brief therapy follows the discussion of the eclectic loop because it requires the therapist to utilize any appropriate technique that will address the acute problem for which the patient has sought therapy.[1] The therapist needs to be comfortable and competent with, and have access to, a wide variety of therapeutic interventions.

Ultra-brief therapy is a circumscribed technique from one to six weeks in duration. The patient is usually seen on a weekly basis—more often only if absolutely necessary—so that there is a set limit of one to six visits. It specifically focuses on an acute event that prompts someone to seek help immediately. Six weeks is not an arbitrary or capricious time frame. Parad, describing the work of Lindeman, Kaplan, and others, showed that the period of enhanced receptivity to change generally extends over a limited time, usually no more than six weeks from the time of the precipitating event or "crisis." Beginning with Lindeman, researchers studied people's responses to significant losses and, based on these responses, developed the foundational theory and techniques of brief therapy.[2] The term *crisis therapy* may be misleading as it conjures images of great drama or trauma. Actually this form of therapy is intended to aid people with *any* acute issue for which they seek immediate attention. For this reason I have coined the term *ultra-brief therapy* to avoid any misleading presumptions induced by the word *crisis*. It focuses on any patient's acute presentation, "I need help right now."

Most people have received emotional help that, although therapeutic, would not be called therapy as such. For example, a person who suddenly has a problem that is sufficiently distressing for him to seek help urgently may go to someone trusted for guidance and counsel. When the help-giver is untrained and unlicensed, the help is not defined as therapy per se. Nevertheless, the person may gain significant therapeutic benefit from the experience.

Ultra-brief therapy takes advantage of a specific and limited receptivity to change created by an acute circumstance: A person losing his job, the death of a loved one, or any other sudden disruptive event. The remarkable willingness to change evoked by the painful event diminishes after six weeks; thereafter other modalities focusing on subacute and chronic circumstances must be employed. Just as heated metal can be reshaped much more readily and with less energy than when it is cold, so too is a person heated by the critical situation more open to change. Once he has cooled off, much greater effort will be needed for him to change—if he remains motivated to do so at all.

As an illustration, let's say an individual refuses to watch his weight or exercise, despite encouragement and/or cajoling by his physicians and loved ones. When he suddenly suffers a heart attack, the situation becomes "hot," and the person feels greatly motivated to lose weight by exercising and eating more appropriate food. He avails himself of all the programs he had previously rebuffed. He is the same person, yet he has suddenly become receptive to changing his behavior because of the serious reality of the situation.

Another example is a wife who has repeatedly threatened to leave her husband if he does not get help with his distressing, erratic behavior. He has troubling and recurrent problems but shows no inclination to change. When the wife actually leaves, the acute threat of permanently losing her may suddenly precipitate the husband's willingness to seek the help he previously had refused.

To further emphasize the importance of the acute, time-specific element in this mode of therapy, picture an individual at a gaming table. A large pile of chips in front of him, he is surrounded by increasing numbers of people who are trying to figure out his winning system. If someone were to suggest that he change the way he plays the game (read: the way he engages in life), his response might vary from at best a polite dismissal to at worst a less-than-friendly gesture. Invariably, the chips begin to flow the other way. His previously winning method now making him a loser, he looks around for the person who offered a different system. Suddenly he is willing to suspend his own technique in favor of one that might work better. A remarkable change in receptivity has occurred. As indicated earlier, research shows that such openness lasts for only a brief time from the onset of the acute precipitating event. Without some sort of immediate, significant intervention, the gambler will probably return to playing the game in the same old way, even though he knows this will no doubt result in further losses.

A charming myth, though linguistically erroneous, has retained its popularity because it so poignantly conveys a truism about critical events. According to the myth, the ideogram for *crisis* in the Mandarin Chinese language is a combination of two other ideograms—one signifying danger, the other opportunity. In this special state, the danger lurks that the acute event will reinforce old patterns, but a great opportunity also avails itself for old behaviors to be readdressed with new solutions. Which path will be taken may be influenced by many factors, among the more favorable ones being too great a pain of staying the same, diminished fear of the new, and certainly the availability of some form of brief therapy.[3] On the other hand, the critical time period may pass without appropriate intervention, and thereby the imminent catalyst for change has been lost. The sudden rattling of our chains often shocks and motivates us into wanting to break free, yet with the passage of time, we find ourselves lulled back into the complacency of tolerating the noise.

Psychopharmacology

Until the 1960s, the use of medication in conjunction with psychoanalysis was anathema. However, in a decision (*Osheroff v. Chestnut Lodge*[4]) that was favorable for a patient who had been hospitalized for long-term analytic treatment of his depression, the court determined that talk therapy alone was below the standard of care. The patient had made remarkable improvement once placed on antidepressants at another treatment facility. This changed the established presumptions that medication interferes with the quality of the therapy work by taking away the pain and suffering that was viewed as motivating the patient to keep exploring his difficulties. The latter position was consistent with the arguments that problems are either nature or nurture, physical or emotional. We have certainly come a long way in the realization that both nature and nurture determine who we become. The brain and the mind are reciprocally interactive.

In the late 1960s, Arnold Mandel and others advocated for the judicious use of appropriate medications for people who were unable to progress in therapy despite every genuine effort to do so.[5] Peter Kramer presented the same thesis in his popular book, *Listening to Prozac,* in which he supports the notion that the patient's inability to make progress in therapy may indicate the need for adjunctive medication.[6]

Studies clearly establish the benefits of medication for people who have definitive symptoms of a major psychiatric disorder: Schizophrenia, depression, bipolar disease, anxiety states, and obsessive-compulsive disorder. Other adjunctively suitable forms of therapy, particularly cognitive behavioral techniques, may be tried in conjunction with medications. These combinations demonstrably increase the benefit to the patient over that of medications alone.[7]

In trying to make changes, patients encounter both anxiety and sadness, and the intensity of these feelings may impede therapeutic progress. In this subtle, gray area, addressed by Mandel and Kramer, where a person's symptoms do not reach the severity of a diagnosable disorder, medication may be most helpful. Therapy falters unless or until medication is employed.

Medication is, of course, not the only alternative when therapy does not progress. Changing the mode of treatment in such situations should also be considered if the current mode's effectiveness has waned. Shifting to another approach can be the equivalent of medication for some people. For example, going from talk therapy to cognitive behavioral therapy in an effort to get around stubborn emotional obstacles has proved effective in reaching solutions not otherwise achievable. The reverse is also true.

A patient may not have the classic diagnostic symptoms, yet his behavior always leads back to reinforcing self-negation, thus defeating the desired goals. Despite all efforts, the eclectic loop of adverse perception —> painful feelings —> symptomatic behavior —> results that negatively reinforce the initial perception seems unbreakable. Empirically utilizing medications for such a patient may be most useful. I term this a *behavioral equivalent of depression,* which may account for the benefit that medications provide when a patient's progress falters.

Couples who fight knowing that it only worsens their relationships, yet acknowledging that it relieves them from internally experiencing painful feelings—paradoxically thereby only increasing their distress—may also be candidates for the use of medication. The "hot potato" of untouchable emotions then cools off enough for them to fight less and express their painful feelings directly, as well as to give them a chance to experience each other in positive ways. The underlying love, caring, and tenderness may come forth as the medication lessens the fear of letting down their rigid defenses against otherwise agonizing emotions.

A woman, the youngest of four children and the only girl in a family that valued only the sons, sought individual therapy. Her brothers and her parents continually belittled her. When she married, the same elements of put-down characterized the husband's devaluing relationship with her. Of course, whom else could she have married? The marriage ended in divorce when the husband decided to pursue other relationships, a typical consequence of his seeing her as having little value. (He will likely repeat the same behavior in his next marriage.) Because of the divorce, the woman had to find work and took a job as an office assistant. At the time, little attention was paid to sexual harassment, and no legal recourse existed. The boss, when not otherwise engaged, thought it his privilege to fondle the woman, which she found disturbing. Although distraught about the advances and feeling contemptuous of the boss, she remained unable to say no or express her disgust. The demeaning behavior represented a consistent element in her family, marriage, and now her job.

Efforts in therapy to explore why she was such a victim and to encourage her to do something about the boss's actions reached an impasse. She understood how her inaction perpetuated self-deprecation, but she was unable to change it. I considered her actions to be the behavioral equivalent of depression and started her on an antidepressant. By the end of the second week on the medication, she was able to grab the boss's hand, pull it away from her, and tell him that his advances were unwelcome. The boss was taken aback but stopped his egregious conduct.

Unfortunately the patient developed significant side effects and had to discontinue the medication. At that time, few alternative drugs without similar side effects existed, in contrast to the variety of agents that are now available in every physician's armamentarium. Two weeks after the patient discontinued the antidepressant, the boss began to fondle her again, and she could no longer say no. Clearly he perceived some subliminal signal that she was once more feeling helpless and unable to defend herself. This case is especially poignant in that it takes antidepressants about two weeks to both take effect and leave the system after discontinuation. It took just those two weeks for the woman to return to the same demeaned state.

In this section, the important interactions between mind and brain and between nature and nurture have been emphasized. Both of these interdependent dyads can be influenced by psychotherapy and the judicious use of medication.

Hypnosis

Hypnosis is another modality that can complement a variety of different therapies.[8] A patient's capacity to utilize hypnosis varies with his ability to concentrate and to use imagery. This ability follows a bell-shaped curve, as do most biological markers. (This does not, however, prove that hypnosis is a biological phenomenon, as I will discuss later.) Some 10 to 15 percent of the population can easily go into a deep trance state. In fact, they probably function in a trance state most of their waking hours without being aware of or knowingly benefiting from this phenomenal gift.

At the other tail of the curve, a similar number of people find it extremely difficult to enter a relaxed state. They may slightly gain from progressive relaxation exercises but cannot go into deep trances. Most of the rest of the population falls under the bell of the curve and can avail themselves of varying benefits. A stage hypnotist skillfully selects those individuals who, by virtue of subtle body language cues, signal that they are already in a trance when asked to come up on stage. The rest is just "show time," although the stage performer would like you to believe otherwise.

This leads to an essential and important fact that must be understood: *All hypnosis is self-hypnosis.* No one can hypnotize another person, notwithstanding legends about Rasputin or Svengali. Unfortunately those who say, "I will/can hypnotize you"—an absolutely false statement—perpetuate this myth. "I will teach you how to use hypnosis, but you are the one who controls how, when, or if you will use it," would be a more accurate assertion. The very word *hypnosis,* derived from the name of the

Greek god of sleep (Hypnos), is in itself misleading. In total contrast to the non-alert state of sleep, the person in a hypnotic trance is in a hyper-alert state, even more so than when normally awake, although with a narrower focus. The only similarity between sleep and trance is the relaxation reached in the trance and that occurring in certain stages of sleep.

No objective, biologic measurements exist to prove that a subject is in a trance, nor is there any definitive proof that hypnosis is a natural biological phenomenon, despite the compellingly similar bell-shaped curve of the distribution of subjects who are able to be hypnotized. An experienced therapist can subjectively identify when a person has entered a trace from the person's increased eye blinks, altered breathing rate, release of muscle tension, and general relaxed physical state. All these signs could be mimicked, however.

Some extraordinary experiments have inferentially shown the trance state as a definitive and special mode of being. For example, hypnotized subjects retain and act on posthypnotic suggestions to a significantly greater degree than do those who only simulate a trance.[9] Even more dramatically, Martin Orne describes a congenitally blind man who was hypnotized and given the suggestion that he would not hear anything but the hypnotherapist's voice. The man showed no reaction when a starter pistol was fired. Yet his EEG (graph of brain waves) showed a spike in his auditory pathway simultaneous with the loud noise.[10]

In another study researchers gave a generally relaxed group of people a suggestion after which the group was compared with a group whose members had first been formally induced into a trance and then given the same suggestion. The researchers subsequently measured the compliance of both groups with the suggestion. The trance group complied in significantly larger numbers and for a longer time than the other group, indicating a greater state of receptivity. These experiments illustrate a very real phenomenon when a person is in a trance as opposed to when he is not, even though biologic markers are lacking.

Hypnosis benefits people in four broad areas:

1. *General ego strengthening.* A suitable subject can be taught to use his powers of concentration and imagery to create a trance state. Realizing through such an experience that he has the natural strength and ability to create a wonderfully relaxed state is in itself an enhancing experience, regardless of whatever problems or diagnosable difficulties exist. The

knowledge that one owns this intrinsic capacity to create a trance is ego strengthening.

2. *Exploration.* Psychodynamically oriented therapies most usefully incorporate this application. It is helpful to think of the trance as allowing the patient to have a seat in the stands, a place to observe his own play on the field. From this position of enhanced alertness, he may see things that he could not otherwise easily recognize. Hypnosis enables the therapist to speak of issues the individual may be reluctant to face or acknowledge in the normal, alert state. Note that anything that can be done with hypnosis can be done without it. The use of hypnosis, however, may shorten the time it takes to reach desired goals.

3. *Habit pattern change.* If the normal alert state is like the light of an ordinary light bulb, then the trance state is like a laser beam. The same "wattage" may be involved with both, but the highly focused hypnotic state allows much greater awareness and intensity while following the various protocols used to help change habitual behavior, such as smoking, overeating, or nail biting.

4. *Pain control.* In this case, the individual is encouraged through assorted hypnotic techniques to modify, objectify, dissociate, distract, or reprocess the experience of pain sensations. With training, subjects can even utilize hypnoanalgesia for surgical procedures. When in a state of intense concentration, such as that of soldiers in battle, good subjects do not experience pain when seriously injured. More prosaically, a person who concentrates on doing some project around the house may later see blood from a significant cut of which he was unaware.

Behavior Leads, Feelings Follow

All therapies endeavor to help patients change symptomatic behavior. The *application* aspect of the four therapeutic components described earlier represents this goal. Very small changes in behaviors precede larger changes in perceptions and feelings.[11] For example, a parent encourages a child to risk tasting a new food that the child is convinced he will not like. If the taste counters the child's negative expectation, the now pleasurable ingestion changes his initial feelings about the food—its color, texture, and taste. Waiting to feel like exercising is another illustration to which most of us can relate. More often than not, it is only after initiating the activity that we feel like doing it.

Even beginning to verbalize conflict-generating feelings becomes a behavioral micro-change that may result in macro-effects. People often fear embarrassment or humiliation if they were to say what they feel. But after doing so, they may exclaim, "Gee, that wasn't as bad as I feared." The absence of the feared reaction encourages further openness.

Referring back to the eclectic loop, when a person risks behaving differently, despite perceptions and feelings to the contrary, and the results prove beneficial, new perceptions and feelings develop. Those feelings in turn promote behavior with positive results, and the momentum builds.

The Importance of Application

The extent of the person's application of what he has learned through the prior stages of confrontation, exploration, and separation determines his Adult's predominant ascendancy over that of his Child. Regardless of the mode of therapy utilized, changing symptomatic behavior and achieving emotional fulfillment are the goals. This necessitates letting go of the maladaptive perceptions, feelings, and behaviors (breaking free) and risking the anxiety of going through zero, which can be an arduous and frightening effort.

Very few adults would turn their car keys over to a small child and then get into the back seat. Disastrous consequences would certainly follow. Yet this is what *unresolved conflict* represents. The pseudo-adult—looking like an adult but controlled by the Child—drives by looking exclusively in the rearview mirror, trying to get away from the past, and ending up running over everyone in his way, who usually do not appreciate that this was unintentional. In attempting to escape from past anguish, we paradoxically recreate it in the present. The Child is always along for the ride in the adult's life, but the kid belongs in the back seat, not behind the wheel.

All the images conjured up—breaking free, going through zero, stepping off the cliff, putting the kid in the back seat and taking the wheel, looking through the windshield and not just through the rear view mirror—represent therapeutic *application,* without which there can be no progress.

Four Stages in Therapy

In addition to the four general components of all therapies described earlier, I have formulated a specific methodology, also divided into four stages, which I find especially useful when working with couples. Together, we explore the "name of the game" that perpetuates their conflicts, how the game is "played" (that is, kept going), and how to quit the game and replace it with something new and different. This approach gives the couple a broad outline of where they are and how to get to where they wish to be.

1. *What is the name of the game?* By this I mean, what is the nature of the problem? What links to the past determine how each person organizes his life and relates intimately with others? What words describe the music of the couple's conflicted dance? Defining their difficulties delineates the shared Need system reflected by a couple's "twinship." We choose our partners because their struggles mesh with ours, and our joint conflict becomes manifested in the marriage. By naming the game, the couple understands the dynamic formulation that describes their *modus operandi*.

2. *How is the game continuing to be played?* What behaviors perpetuate the very thing the couple wishes to be different? In other words, how are they continuing to express what they once Needed rather than what they now Want?

3. *Quitting.* Quitting, similar to what was discussed about the separation and application phases of therapy, entails applying what has been learned in the two prior stages. This is a major step for most couples because regardless of their ages or how long they have been married, stopping behaviors learned in childhood that perpetuate problems symbolizes emotionally leaving home for the first time. Never before have they risked going through zero by breaking away from their Need chains in favor of having what they Want. A great deal of sadness, anxiety, and fear may accompany this process. A person may grieve the loss of what might have been but never will be. Recall the man's dream of seeing himself as the boy he once was in a gutter.

4. *Doing something new and different.* Although clearing out the old is necessary for creating space for the new, it is the beginning, not the end. *The absence of the negative is not the same as the presence of the positive.* The

couple now has the opportunity to actually experience—not just fantasize about—what they Want, or desire, in their relationship. They have to be patient and diligent, however. Doing something truly new and different feels awkward, stilted, unnatural, and even mechanical. This is to be expected. Just as when learning to dance, it is a clumsy endeavor; not until the behavior is well practiced does it come off as smooth and natural.

Communication: Artistic or Autistic

The communication of thoughts and feelings that lead to understanding is an artistic expression. This is true for any form of communication, be it written, verbal, or in any other art form. A message is sent, and a message is received. The intended communication is understood. If a message is sent but cannot be understood, the communication is autistic. (This communication is psychologically based and not to be confused with the diagnosable condition of autism.)

We often describe thoughts, behaviors, and feelings to which we simply cannot relate as "crazy." Usually this is because we do not comprehend any meaning in the message and therefore may dismiss it as irrational. How vastly different is our experience of the other person when we do get the meaning in his message. With understanding, autistic communication becomes artistic, and the person no longer seems crazy.

When I was a resident in psychiatry, one of my supervisors, Norbert I. Rieger, taught me something enormously valuable about the power of understanding. In discussing a patient who exhibited psychotic thinking, I had great difficulty making the diagnosis. Though recognizing the psychotic symptoms, I was uncomfortable attaching the corresponding label that unquestionably applied. Rieger helped me understand my reticence by explaining that the patient had let me into his secret world, which was populated by all kinds of special creatures. In spite of his psychotic disorder, he had described each of these creatures and the role they played in his life in a manner easy for me to understand. That made the difference between communicating in an *artistic* versus an *autistic* way. It is only when a communication is not understood that it is autistic. Once we comprehend the message, it becomes artistic. This is true in the arts as well. Does a painting or an expression in any of the arts speak to us? If so, then we understand the work as artistic.

I have made this point before, but because I believe it is important I am repeating it here: Feeling understood is a profound experience, as is that of understanding the feelings of another. People describe it as similar to loving or feeling loved. Obviously in adversarial relationships in which communication is oriented toward attacking and defending—not understanding—this cannot occur.

We often frame our conflicts in terms of winners and losers, as though the participants are in a courtroom vying for the winning position. This is the *power play* mode of relating. Notwithstanding their sometimes awful behaviors, couples who adopt adversarial postures may actually love their mates, but the intensity of the old, unresolved issues, perpetrated in the present, obscures this love and prevents them from engaging in the *love play* mode. Like a garden overgrown with weeds, the flowers cannot be seen. It is imperative for the therapist to facilitate constructive communication that centers on understanding and not on judging.

A Communication Guide

In any relationship—but especially in intimate ones—it is important to communicate in a positive, friendly way that does not alienate or antagonize the other person. Modifying Thomas Gordon's "I Message"[12] concept of communicating feelings, I emphasize three major components that I often encourage patients to use as a guide:

1. *Having a good-faith assumption.* "My partner is not out to get me and is not willfully, malignantly, maliciously, or consciously attempting to hurt me by what he says or does." (If—in the highly unlikely case—he actually is, this must be addressed first and takes precedence over any other issue.) "If I feel hurt, there must be some important reason why my partner said what he said or did what he did. My partner is responsible for his actions or statements, but I am responsible for how I feel in response. No one can make me feel what I feel." (Recall the 7-Eleven story in Chapter Five.)

2. *Understanding.* "My task's operating principle is to try to understand— not judge—why my partner did what he did or said what he said. If I judge, I am being adversarial and will not likely understand. If I understand, I am being an ally and likely won't find judging necessary. At all times it is essential that I respect my partner and myself while expressing my feelings."

3. *Identifying feelings.* Anger is never a primary emotion and has no ultimate value in an intimate relationship. "If I experience anger, I am

hiding the more intimate and vulnerable primary feelings that I must identify, experience, and express. If I don't, I'll just be going down an emotional blind alley. If I can substitute 'I think' for 'I feel' and what I say still makes sense, then I am verbalizing a thought and not a feeling. If I use 'that,' 'like,' or 'you" following either 'I think' or 'I feel,' then I am probably giving voice to a thought—often accusatory in nature—and not sharing my feelings."

In summary:

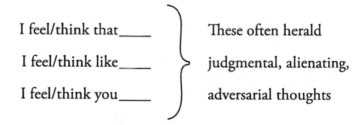

I feel/think that____	These often herald
I feel/think like____	judgmental, alienating,
I feel/think you____	adversarial thoughts

Caveat: Expressions of thoughts or opinions can always be disputed. Everyone can perceive situational facts differently; we can even agree to disagree about facts. But when feelings are honestly expressed, they are never judgments; they are always valid, and therefore they cannot be refuted. This is true because those feelings reside totally in the owner's emotional domain. Although they may not entirely have to do with the present, it is important to understand what perceptions in the present may have evoked those feelings.

Using this guide we can communicate *any* feelings. Because emotions or feelings have to do with ourselves and can never be judgments or attacks on others, there should be no reason to withhold their expression nor any need for "walking on eggshells" with anyone who is interested in listening and trying to understand. Being able to freely express our deepest feelings enhances the intimacy of our relationships.

A Guide for Listening

When the listener finds expressed feelings painful and difficult to hear, he often steps in and tries to negate the feelings. "Oh, you don't have to feel that way." "It's silly for you to feel that." "How could you possibly feel that?" "Your feelings make no sense." This may even represent a well-intentioned attempt to solve the other person's problem and make him feel better, or it may be an effort to avoid feeling uncomfortable oneself.

In any relationship, the experience of actually being listened to makes an enormous difference in our perception of the relationship's value. The guide for communication outlined above enables us to express our feelings and engage in intimate dialogue. However crucial verbalizing emotions may be it is essential to have a guide for listening as well. This poem, which I have considerably modified from its anonymous source, illustrates the potential pitfalls of giving advice when not asked and the rewards of good listening:

Please Just Listen

When I ask you to listen to me and instead you start giving advice,
you have not done what I asked, nor heard what I desire.
When I ask you to listen to me and you begin to tell me
why I shouldn't feel what I am feeling,
you are trampling on my feelings.
When I ask you to listen to me, and you feel you have to do
something to solve my problems,
you have failed me—strange as that may seem.
Listen, please!
All I ask is that you listen. Not talk, nor "do"—just hear me.
Advice is cheap when not asked for. Fifty cents gets me "Dear Abby"
and the astrology forecasts in the same paper.
I can do that for myself.
I am not helpless. Maybe discouraged or faltering—but not helpless.
When you do something for me that I can and must to do for myself,
you contribute to my seeming fearful, weak, or inadequate.
I may feel these things. Don't act as though my feelings are facts.
When you accept that I feel what I feel, no matter how irrational
it seems, I can quit trying to convince you and instead begin to
understand what is behind what I am saying and doing—to what I
am feeling.
When that is clear, chances are so will the answers be, and I won't
need advice -
Or I will then be ready to hear it!
Perhaps that is why for some people prayer works.

God is mute and doesn't give advice or try to fix what we must do
ourselves.
So please listen, just hear me.
And if you wish to speak, let's plan on your turn.
I promise I will listen, too.

Utilizing these guides—one for talking and one for listening—will enrich our emotionally intimate communications with significant others.

Fairy Tales

Freud spoke of dreams as the "royal road to the unconscious."[13] I am deeply indebted to Berne for his elegant description of the way fairy tales reveal people's conflicted narratives.[14] Fairy tales—as well as other classic literature, myths, and even some song lyrics—express the core of important, universal emotional struggles.[15]

The following are just a few examples of the themes that give voice to common conflicts with which most people can identify, which allows the stories to survive from generation to generation:

- *Sleeping Beauty*: the competitive mother

- *Hansel and Gretel*: the weak father and wicked "stepmother" who abandon their children

- *Heidi:* the longing for home

- *Jack and the Bean Stalk*: a young man's struggle to be potent and valued by the significant woman in his life, even when the shadow of father looms large

- *Cinderella*: feeling like a stepchild, abused by siblings, having a cruel (step-) mother and impotent father, and fantasies of rescue by a handsome prince

Sometimes when I am trying to understand the fundamental nature of a patient's difficulties or want to emphasize an emotional theme, I will ask the patient to indulge me as follows: "Please tell me the first thing that comes to your mind when you think of a fairy tale" (or favorite story, poem, song lyrics, etc.). Invariably the patient will come up with exactly the story line that best describes his conflicts in a basic, straightforward, and clear way. At times he does not even recall the story, only the name of the tale. Nevertheless after he and I reread it we usually find that it precisely represents the crux of his conflicts.

I have shared this idea with therapists-in-training over the years, and they too have been impressed with how succinctly the tales, stories, lyrics, and so forth capture the nature of the struggles of patients. Always in awe of how keenly our minds work in seeking ways to express important issues, I often assure patients, "You can trust your mind to take you to that which requires your attention—if you just don't try to stop it from doing the job."

Simple Not Simplistic

I have come to believe that human conflict is simple to understand and describe. As complex as we are as human beings, it is nonetheless a complexity made of simple stuff. The idea of a simple theme may seem simplistic to the reader. But I caution that there is a very important difference between simple and simplistic.

For example, look at the enormous intricacies of some spiders' webs as a metaphor for human conflict: Fantastic geometric shapes of great design woven essentially from a single, extruded strand of spider silk. There may be different types of silk in the spider's repertoire, but the insect weaves only one kind at a time. So it is with human beings; we weave complex designs by extruding a simple thread of conflict. The therapist finds the thread and unravels the weave through his dynamic formulation, spoken of in chapter six, which will be further illustrated in the discussion of clinical cases in chapter nine.

Another metaphor makes the same point. In spite of the enormous magnitude of the universe as we know it, physicists have sought a simple and elegant "theory of everything," a single theory that unites gravity, electromagnetism, the weak forces, and the strong forces. A hotly debated and controversial contender for this unified concept is the simple, albeit mind-bending, idea of string theory.[16] If this theory were to ultimately prove true, the entirety of the universe would derive from the vibrations of infinitesimally small strings. The nuclear age in which we live could be viewed as emanating from a simple equation: $E = mc^2$. For human emotional conflict, the dynamic formulation describes a unitary theme—

the simple thread of a person's conflict woven into complex, multitudinous patterns of woe.

It is important to appreciate that our struggles, no matter how profoundly manifested, are made of deep but simple issues, not to be confused with or dismissed as superficially simplistic.

Elements Contained in All Therapies

For all their differences, the therapies described in this and the previous chapter have several fundamental commonalities. Jerome Frank describes some of these as *positive expectations, the placebo effect, healing rituals, positive transference,* and *catharsis.*[17] Karl Menninger said that a therapist ultimately provides patients only with "love and hope."[18] By love he meant Rollo May's definition of love: The willingness to contribute to another's healthy growth.[19]

All competent therapists offer patients hope, interest, trust, and respect. These qualities are independent of any specific theory or treatment technique and help the patient break free from old constraints and risk feeling adrift in order to move from the negative in his life to the positive. My emphasis has been on talk therapy and the importance of verbalizing and understanding the nature of our struggles to change. The other techniques mentioned may be equally useful in helping people grow as long as those procedures are engaged in ethically and competently.

Chaos Theory

I would like to share some thoughts about a concept borrowed from mathematics known as *chaos theory.*[20] Its application to medicine in general and psychiatry in particular is in its infancy. A more complete discussion of the topic would deserve at least a separate chapter or preferably a book of its own. Suffice it for me to briefly and simply describe some ideas derived from chaos theory that I find useful in thinking about psychotherapy.

Human beings are nonlinear (our reactions are dynamic and variable, not static), open (we continuously react with the environment) systems. Examples of other such systems that we encounter daily are weather patterns, organizational behavior, cardiac function, and shifts in public opinion. Chaos/complexity theory provides an understanding of how new activity patterns can develop in prompt response to either familiar or completely novel stimuli. It has been shown that aging leads to a loss of complexity/chaos in the functioning of healthy organs. This results in a diminished ability to respond to stress. As the organs' capacity for randomness decreases, fixed response patterns increase.

The greater the degree of flexibility a system has, the greater its ability to adapt to changing circumstances. Having a steady, totally predictable heart rate, for instance, would lead to an inability to respond to changing circumstances, such as exercise or fright, and ultimately result in a failure of heart function. The same applies to brain wave patterns and hormonal release cycles. The more fixed they are, the more fragile they are. This means the more we can accept the unpredictable, the better our adaptive ability to survive and thrive.

Chaos theory is a balancing act between a totally deterministic world in which there would be no choices and a completely random world in which predictability of any kind would be impossible, as there would be no way of making reasoned decisions. Instead, these open, nonlinear, and—for our purposes—human systems depend on initial conditions that are magnified in unpredictable ways. For example, small events in a child's life take on larger significance in unpredictable ways as the child grows. This intensifying and enlarging impact that grows from a simple start has been called the *butterfly effect*. It proposes that the flapping of a butterfly's wings in Brazil could ultimately result in a tornado in Texas.[21] Essentially this means that small starting circumstances can have profound ultimate effects.

In human history, major events can often be traced to the subsequent magnifications of initial, ultimately unpredictable behaviors of single personalities. Modern examples are Eisenhower's choosing the date for the D-Day invasion, Hitler's neglecting to fully fortify a landing beach, George H. W. Bush's declining to invade Iraq, or George W. Bush's doing so—simple decisions with profound and unpredictable consequences.

If the behaviors in such an open, nonlinear system are neither random nor determined, how are they organized? Chaos theory postulates that they are organized around *strange attractors*.[22] Human decision-making has to account for many assumptions and implications that could become paralyzing. The strange attractor helps us organize our thoughts and behaviors. For example, a strange attractor could be our religious or political belief systems. In the terms used in this book the organizing strange attractor could be our Child Needs.

Living in the present has a special meaning in chaos theory. "Now" is the edge of a transitional state in which all choices are open. In each moment we have the opportunity to make choices that will determine the next step we take and the life we will live. As when coming to a fork in the road, each such moment is a point of choice whereby a new strange attractor has an opportunity to operate, and the human being can adapt and potentially continue to grow. It allows for the development of *order out of chaos*. For reasons related to the self-organizing features of living systems—namely, the potential adaptability to new circumstances—Heinz von Foerster proposed that we call ourselves not human beings but human *becomings*.[23]

Here I return to the Bible once more without any necessary reference to theological beliefs. Moses (Exodus 3:14) asks the voice in the burning bush to state his name. Using the future tense, God replies, "I will be who I will be," or according to another interpretation, "I will be what tomorrow demands." It is fascinating to reflect on God's supposed answer as representing the capacity to meet new circumstances with complete adaptability. This response clearly implies an evolving, dynamic character to the deity—not a static, fixed, rigid one. What a terrific model to emulate.

I find chaos theory valuable for the theses I have presented because it speaks to the importance of continually finding a place between rigidity, with no capacity to adapt, and randomness, with nothing to adapt to. Because of the emotional need for familiarity and predictability, the Child's beliefs cause fixed behavior patterns that can limit the adult's capacity to respond freely to new circumstances. The Need to keep today like yesterday prevents a person from living in the now. The omnipresent opportunities to *become* are denied and lost. The consequence is less capacity to adapt, more rigidity, and greater fragility. Choice is sacrificed.

The more we risk letting go of stultifying certainty to allow new constructs, the better the outcome. The relief of symptoms corresponds to the freedom to choose and adapt to new and healthy attractors. Translating this into the terms used earlier, relief comes from breaking free of fixed Needs in order to adaptively implement Wants. The imperative lies in recognizing and utilizing the essential and continuing existence of choice at every critical time in life.

CHAPTER EIGHT

Anger, Guilt, and Projective Identification

In this chapter I will expand on the concepts of anger, guilt, and projective identification to which I have alluded in the previous chapters. Clarifying my use of these terms will facilitate the understanding of the clinical material presented in chapter nine. The common thread in the three phenomena is that they are mechanisms that maintain, rather than resolve, emotional conflicts.

Anger

Anger is a fundamental emotional state that had great evolutionary value in primordial times. Survival depended on taking action in response to a perceived threat—either fight or flee. Fear, once converted to anger, prompted a fight response, whereas its direct expression fueled flight. Either option involves considerable physical exertion.

Willard Gaylin has described how these responses have become maladaptive because we now live in crowded urban and suburban centers and not on the savanna.[1] Every community's police blotter attests to the destructive outcome resulting from these primordial defensive displays. Long gone, I hope, are the days when getting a patient to express anger was thought the end goal of therapy. Gone also is the padded bat called a *bataka* with which the patient could pound out these angry feelings. For some people, expressing anger may be a starting point for the expression of feelings, but at best, it must be a transient phase.

The realization that anger is always a secondary emotion and never a primary one makes such expression even more dysfunctional. Imagine what you would feel if I were to walk over and stomp on your foot. Your first sensation would be to feel *pain*. But your first expression might well be rage, especially if you perceived my stomping as a deliberate act. On the other hand, you might express simple irritation if you ascribed to my action innocent clumsiness. Whatever the case, anger, irritation, or annoyance would be secondary to the primary experience of pain.

This is not to imply that anger is totally without value. Having access to such an emotion might prove handy when dealing with difficult people in some societal circumstances. The conundrum is that expressing anger generally serves only to beget more anger.

Love involves risk. The more intimate we desire a relationship to be, the less appropriate our expression of anger is. Anger shields the "soft underbelly" feelings of loss, pain, grief, helplessness, or fear. Therefore anger is a way of *avoiding* risk and *preventing* intimacy. When we dare to be intimate, we have no absolute certainty of safety, only a reasonable chance for love.

We must not hide behind a shield and then wonder why we cannot get close to others. The realization that the adult's vulnerability no longer equates with the child's helplessness makes letting go of the anger defense possible. Any relationship sacrifices intimacy and understanding when anger is its predominant mode of expression. Think of anger as a suit of armor. How cozy can one get with someone dressed in armor? Safety is achieved, but intimacy is lost.

I have stressed the importance of understanding the phenomenon of anger to illustrate how easily it keeps us from acknowledging our primary feelings. Its ubiquitous use defends against owning and resolving feelings that often stem from old conflicts. By clinging to those conflicts, we hold onto the past with its once perceived safety to avoid the fear of change.

Guilt

Guilt is often associated with shame and considered a similar emotion, but there is a significant distinction between the two. Shame is a painful feeling evoked when we believe that we have fallen below some group norm or standard. It no doubt evolved in early human development as an important way to maintain a tribe's social cohesiveness and control of its members. Though shame is a powerful emotion, I propose that guilt is not. Rather, I suggest that guilt is a *mechanism allowing for experiencing connectedness*. Guilt certainly exists as a societal phenomenon: Break the law, and one is judged guilty. How we may feel about such a judgment puts us back into the emotional realm, including that of shame. I like using Freud's "Mourning and Melancholia," arguably the beginning of object relations theory according to Fairbairn, as a way of illustrating this guilt concept as a mechanism.

Fairbairn proposed that the real parents have both good and bad aspects and that the child will split off and internalize the bad. He gains the advantage of now having all-good, idealized parents while he, the child, contains the bad. An expensive maneuver, it costs the child diminished ego strength, or mental energy, keeping the awareness of the origin of the bad feelings submerged.[2]

Psychodynamically oriented therapists have great interest in focusing on the patient's relationships with his parents, not to make them out to be the bad ones but to help the patient see his significant others as real people with both good and bad characteristics. When he can do so, he can regain the ego strength that he expended in maintaining the idealization; as a result, the self can also be seen as real and whole.

I have diagrammed Freud's ideas from "Mourning and Melancholia" to illustrate the guilt bond established by a survivor who had a conflicted relationship with a deceased significant other. Each of the real persons is "split" into unrealistic perceptions of an all-good significant other (the deceased) and the bad self (the grieving survivor). The real aspects of self and other are submerged into either an unconscious or a subliminal (barely aware) state. Resolution begins when the subliminal or unconscious is made conscious.

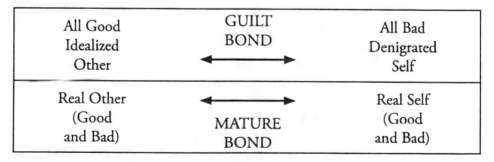

Figure 8-1 Guilt and Mature Bonds

Because we will all experience the death of a significant person in our lives, I want to expand further on the grieving process and what commonly interferes with healthy mourning. When confronted with the death of a significant other, one may idealize that person. Potential problems ensue because idealization blocks the recognition of the deceased as a real person who had both good and bad characteristics. The grieving survivor may begin to experience himself as diminished, especially in relation to the now-idealized deceased. Although differing stages of grief have been postulated[3], I am suggesting that the persistence of idealization impedes the grieving process.

When the survivor idealizes the deceased and consequently denigrates himself he establishes a connection with the deceased through a guilt bond. Why would one engage in such a maneuver? Because this mechanism allows the survivor to avoid experiencing the terrible pain of the void created by the death. The greater the unexplored conflict between the deceased and the survivor, the greater the propensity for aberrant grieving. Death eliminates any hope of an improved relationship. The deceased is gone, but a lot of unfinished business remains. How can one possibly let go?

Eulogies demonstrate the prevalence of such idealization. The comments often bear little resemblance to the person the deceased really was. Sometimes the recollections are so distorted that it is difficult to recognize the individual who died. Here is a humorous refection on this phenomenon. How do you tell the difference between a testimonial and a eulogy? In the former, there is at least one person who believes what is being said.

Grieving survivors may lament not having been kinder or more considerate toward the deceased. If they evade reflecting on what in the relationship led them to behave the way they did, the deceased will get a free pass. Freud cautioned that melancholia would follow incomplete mourning. The goal of grief work is for the grieving person to acknowledge that the deceased was a real person, refrain from idealizing him, and process the feelings created by the void. The guilt connection functions to avoid experiencing the loss. The cost is self-denigration. The consequence is melancholia.

Consider this common illustration: An elderly mother, bitter and constantly complaining, was placed in a nursing home. With aging, vinegar poured into a bottle does not become fine wine. When the adult children and grandchildren visited, she harangued them and complained that they never came to see her. As she became increasingly unpleasant, her children avoided going to visit her, instead encouraging the grandchildren to visit their grandmother. Without awareness, the adult children, avoiding the painful emptiness of their relationship with her, began developing a guilt bond, which they displaced onto the grandchildren (a "ticking emotional bomb"). The parents suggested that the (now) bad-for-not-visiting grandchildren could expiate their own guilt through their visits. "Why don't you ever go and see Granny?" they exhorted. "She's so lonely and would really like to see you." When the inevitable call came that grandmother had died, an outpouring of self-recriminations by the parents followed (the "bomb" explodes). "Why didn't we go more often? How difficult would it have been to go every Sunday? We feel so guilty for how we treated her." It is important to recognize this common scenario and to prevent guilt cycles from developing.

In healthy grieving, the survivors are encouraged to acknowledge that Grandma was often a difficult person, unable to appreciate efforts made on her behalf. Her demeanor does not make her bad but rather troubled. Recognizing that Grandma struggled with unsolved problems from her own past helps the survivors change their attitude. At the same time it is important to honor her good side, no matter how minuscule. She was a real person, good and bad, and therefore so too are the survivors. For mourning to be complete we have to accept the void created by the loss, experience the sadness, rejoice in what was positive, and grieve for what was not.

A young woman seeking therapy because of her abruptly changed behavior provides another example of how guilt may be used to avoid feelings of loss. She was barely twenty-one years old and had been married for only a short time to a twenty-four-year-old man. They were deeply in love and looked forward to having a family and a long life together. The husband was an ardent marathon runner in great physical shape except for an unknown heart rhythm abnormality. While running one day, he suddenly dropped dead. The wife was devastated. She was raised with good moral standards and had always been appropriate and mature in her relationships. In response to this dreadful event, she began to frequent bars, pick up strange men, and take them home for sex. Her behavior shocked and distressed her enough that she came to therapy.

It quickly became evident that this woman attempted to avoid dealing with the loss of her beloved husband by magnifying the perception of how good he was, especially in contrast to how badly she now behaved. "I feel so guilty. John would be furious with me." She subsequently acknowledged her fantasy that he would somehow learn of her sordid behavior, and the more badly she behaved, the greater the possibility that John would return to both castigate and rescue her. This woman had no psychotic disorder or any psychiatric history; she was simply trying desperately to avoid having to face never seeing her beloved again.

For meaningful completion of mourning, we must avoid the trap of maintaining contact through a guilt bond. A patient expressed admiration for her cousin's marriage, wishing that her own could be as satisfactory. I could not tell if she admired a real or an idealized relationship. Suddenly and unexpectedly, the cousin's husband died. The patient related how people came to the home to pay their respects after the funeral. It was winter, and snow had become trapped against the wooden front door and the storm door, causing the wood to swell and stick. The widow had repeatedly complained about this to her husband before his death. As she now saw people out and the door again stuck, she spontaneously said, "Damn it, couldn't you have fixed this before you died?" I then knew the patient's description of her cousin's relationship was accurate and not idealized. The widow comfortably recognized her husband as a real person who often procrastinated in doing household tasks. Her love for him acknowledged his foibles as well as his strengths.

The guilt bond in dealing with a deceased person also occurs in conflicted interactions with still-living significant others. If in a current relationship we dread acknowledging the realness—good and bad—of the vital other, then the potential for guilt bonding exists. The bond serves the same function: Fending off feeling the absence of any healthy connection. We may even engage in self-denigrating behaviors that reinforce our notion of being bad, thereby justifying our guilty feelings. The death of a significant other with whom unresolved conflicts exist creates a profound feeling of loss within us. A poor ongoing relationship generates a similar void: The emptiness caused by the unfulfilled desire for a better relationship. In either situation, by connecting through a guilt mechanism, we attempt to ignore the sadness about not having—or having had—a meaningful relationship.

The adolescent who engages in delinquent behavior and the spouse who has extramarital affairs and then feels guilty in relationship to the vital other—parent or spouse—illustrates this phenomenon. Both avoid confronting the distress that they experience in their relationships. The acting-out behavior speaks to an existing problem but does so in a way that deflects attention from the salient question: What is wrong with the parenting of an adolescent who engages in delinquent behavior? What is the problem in the marriage that drives a spouse to have affairs? These questions must be addressed if there is to be any change. Doing so, however, threatens the nature of the relationship, because facing the problems forces a shift in the interactions that could lead to the loss of the relationship. The person must accept this uncertainty for the relationship to improve. If both parties do not commit to solving the difficulties, the relationship may end.

And so the potential void looms, anticipated with dread. This is the challenge of breaking free. Instead of taking that chance and facing zero, the person establishes and maintains a guilt bond as a substitute for the emptiness he feels. Masterson's "tie that binds" concept expresses the same idea of having to let go in order to grow,[4] but this requires that the person tolerate the apprehension of the possible disconnection. Without acknowledging his fears about risking the challenge, nothing can change, and guilt remains the desperate connection to the idealized significant other.

I have described the guilt bond from the perspective of the denigrated self relating to the idealized other. Looking at the relationship from the opposite vantage point, the idealized person may connect with a *power bond* that keeps the guilty other in an inferior position. As long as the "bad other" continues connecting with guilt, the power-bonded, all-good person does not jeopardize losing the relationship and may not be motivated to make any changes. Take for example the husband who belittles his spouse, both privately and in public. The wife accepts this denigration, feels guilty for being a lesser person, and continues allowing herself to idealize her husband. She bonds through guilt, he with power. When the guilty one dies, the survivor may maintain his power connection by speaking only ill of the dead.

Several decades ago, ferment began in the American Catholic Church that further describes this phenomenon, although on a much larger scale. I cite this with full respect for the principles of the faith and its adherents and with the recognition that the description may apply equally well to other organized institutions. When the church is viewed as all good and the parishioners as primarily bad or sinful, a power-guilt bond is established. Liberal Catholic theologians promulgated the idea that the institution, as with any human endeavor, was not all good. They saw that aspects of the Church were functionally bad, as painfully evident by the revelations of sexual abuse by priests. In the view of these theologians, the organization should not be idealized but rather seen as real and requiring change. Simultaneously, parishioners recognized that they had something of value to offer the institution. Once we appreciate this real perception of self and other—good and bad—we no longer connect with guilt. But then we must face the void that is left when we disconnect, as well as the opportunity to forge a new and different relationship of mutuality. Looking in from the outside, this seems to be one aspect of the contemporary struggle with which both Church and parishioners are engaged. (In citing this example, I refer only to the psychological dimensions of the organizational interaction and the parallels that exist in any other human relationship.)

Projective Identification

The third phenomenon, *projective identification*,[5] is a common and troublesome way of communicating feelings through behavior. The trouble begins when we try to be in two emotional places at the same time. How can we let another person know what we feel while simultaneously defending against feared consequences? Our guard remains up, yet we desire to communicate.

To illustrate this, let's say that I am feeling terrified and urgently want you to know what I feel so you can comfort and help me. On the other hand, I am uncertain how you will respond to my exposing such profound feelings. I feel conflicted by wanting to be intimate and trying to be safe at the same time. How can I solve this dilemma?

I can behave in such a way that my actions induce in you the very feeling I am trying to express. How might I do this? I could take a gun and point it at you, terrifying you. Now you feel *exactly* what I am feeling. But have I really succeeded in communicating my feelings to you? Hardly! Instead of being able to recognize that what you experience is actually an important message from me, you are only aware of your own terror of having someone pointing a gun at you.

This simple example describes an all-too-common mode by which people in close relationships try to negotiate between Wanting to be intimate and Needing to be safe. Their behavior aims at creating a parallel feeling in the other person. "I feel hurt by your cheating, but I'll be damned if I'll let you know the impact it has on me. Instead I'm going to cheat on you. Then when you find out you'll know just how I feel."

Here is another example. Parents are terrified when their child does not return from school on time. They search with no success. Out of complete desperation they finally call the police. The parents begin to have all kinds of fearful images of what might have happened and experience profound feelings of helplessness along with terror. Amid the crowd of friends and neighbors gathered to help and comfort them comes forth their carefree child, obviously perfectly healthy and unaware of any problem. He had simply seen a frog and, mesmerized, followed it until it disappeared in the darkness. What do the parents do? The great relief they initially felt suddenly turns to rage at the child. They hold him responsible for their feelings of fear and helplessness. Then they launch a punitive attack on him, and lo and behold, the poor kid now experiences the overwhelming terror and profound helplessness the parents had felt.

Acting out deep feelings, instead of risking the vulnerability of communicating such feelings in words, leaves the other(s) trying to figure out just what the action means. The nature of the behavior used to transmit uncomfortable feelings is often aggressive. The recipient likely becomes reasonably defensive in response. By acting out, the person attempts to be both safe and intimate at the same time—in other words, he tries to stay chained to old postures while wishing to be free. Such communicating defeats his desire to be close, creating even greater distance. It is a bit like kids hitting each other in the attempt to express themselves. Sharing vulnerable feelings directly accomplishes the goal more effectively and preferably—especially so in valued relationships.

As the recipient of such a communication, one can "decode" the message by monitoring one's own internal, emotional response *without* becoming defensive. If a child tells his parents, "I hate you," a healthy response would be, "Wow, that feels painful. Are you trying to tell me how much you are hurting?"

Integration

All the metaphors I have used to discuss change—such as falling off a cliff, becoming an orphan when letting go of unhealthy familiar/familial behavior, and risking going through zero—are attempts to vivify how intense the struggle to break old chains can be. Freud proposed that people change only when the pain of the present circumstances becomes intolerable, or when the fear of the new situation diminishes enough to allow one to explore it. This reflects the power of the emotions of fear and pain. The awareness that the adult always has choices facilitates a person's ability to change.

Up to this point, I have presented various ideas—some new and different, some old and familiar. Understanding how emotional conflicts may cause our earliest relationships' unique characteristics to develop and the reasons for their distressing persistence contributes to a more productive therapy relationship. The composite case vignettes that follow make the major points clearer and, we hope, more useful to the reader.

CHAPTER NINE

Clinical Vignettes

As diverse as cultures, customs, and mores may be, there is a fundamental sameness to all human beings. The desire to love and be loved and to feel safe, nurtured, supported, comforted, and encouraged remains the essence of who we are, no matter where we may live. So too is there a sameness in the way we defend against the pain of having such desires thwarted.

Clinical illustrations offer a glimpse into other people's struggles to resolve conflicts. We identify with some of those problems, which may help us solve our own. Others disturb us, because we cannot accept our own potential for having to struggle with the same issues.

Aside from important biological and genetic factors, the degree of propensity for similar issues ultimately distinguishes one person who has diagnosable symptoms from one who does not. For example, although everyone who anticipates giving a speech feels some apprehension, for some, the intensity of these feelings may reach a level consistent with diagnosable social phobia. Similarly, feelings of insecurity are common to all people and vary depending upon the situation. A cartoonist depicts this quintessential commonality in a sketch showing a large number of people at a bus stop. They are drawn to represent a cross section of society—businesspeople, teenagers, women shoppers, children, the elderly, and so on. A large bubble shows what they are all thinking: "I wonder if anyone else feels as insecure as I do?"

We share common behavioral capacities as well, even the potential

149

for those behaviors that we judge incomprehensible and inhumane. Both Mitscherlich[1] and Lifton[2] have documented how ordinary doctors were induced to perpetrate unspeakable crimes as Nazi physicians. Goethe's comment, "There is no crime of which I do not deem myself capable,"[3] captures this human commonality. If we deny our own capacity to commit horrific acts, we blind ourselves to how easily that denial could pave the way, through the absence of vigilance, for us to perpetuate such acts.

Take, for example, the abhorrence of torture. Prominent governmental officials have proclaimed, "The United States does not engage in torture," as if such a statement, coupled with our historical values, makes Americans' torture of prisoners utterly inconceivable. Hannah Arendt described the stupefying "banality of evil" associated with committing horrible deeds.[4] The extermination of people, purged of its killing connotation, becomes "ethnic cleansing" and almost business as usual for some regimes. If we say that only "nonhumans" are capable of such inhumane acts, then we ignore our universality. When we relegate perpetrators of heinous acts to a subhuman category, we paradoxically commit the inhumane. If we laugh at the plight of others, we act as though we are superior to them. When we refer to fellow human beings as wops, mics, heimies, chinks, scum, queers, whities, or gooks—to name just a few derogatory terms—we attempt to assassinate, figuratively if not literally, the humanity of those so denigrated. Displacing our own inferior feelings onto others allows us to feel superior—as long as we keep the lesser others in their place. Of course it follows, according to such logic, that superior people never do inferior things.

An inexcusable, if milder, example of denigration occurs when a group of therapists viewing a videotape of a patient's interview laugh at some foible the patient reveals. Would they laugh if the patient were present in the room? Such conduct should not be tolerated. This is very different from laughing *with* the patient. Obviously some in attendance identify with something the patient says or does and release their uncomfortable tension through laughter. Nevertheless, as therapists, we ought to recognize our resonance with the messenger rather than ever mocking him *in absentia*.

I present the following case illustrations in the spirit that the story of one is the story of all. They are modified in certain details to maintain confidentiality, but without sacrificing the essence of the patterns I wish to illuminate. In each example, those individuals described, like all of us, implicitly hold onto their maladaptive behaviors—the Need bonds—to subvert facing the void of change. In the process of doing so, they sacrifice what they say they Want.

When I begin therapy with a new patient, I inquire about his family of origin by simply saying, "Tell me about your family." I want to know with whom the patient will start, whom he will include, and most important, whom he may leave out. If necessary, I may then be more specific by saying, "Using words to paint a picture, describe your parents for me." When the patient has drawn a picture of each parent, I ask about the relationship between the parents—Are there siblings? What are they like? What is the birth order? What is the history of their relationships?—and so on as I gather the pertinent information about the family and their relationships.

When listening to case presentations at conferences or in supervising trainees, I imagine a "hat tree" upon which I hang each piece of information. This allows me to recognize which hooks are filled and in what order and which are still empty. I can then start to hypothesize about the information presented and why it was done in a particular fashion, thereby beginning my dynamic formulation.

William Osler, a famous physician of the early twentieth century, said, "Listen to the patient, he is telling you the diagnosis."[5] Though we now have at our disposal sophisticated lab tests and diagnostic equipment, this adage remains important in treating patients. In psychotherapy it is vital. People will use precisely the words that best describe who the actors are in their lives and how they act.

When working with a couple, I may also ask each spouse if he or she wishes to add anything to the descriptions. A partner's view may clarify, add to, or modify the emphasis in the picture provided by the first spouse. Occasionally it turns out to be the first time the significant other has ever heard some important, intimate, or emotional detail about the partner or his family.

Initials Tell All

Emma T. is an attractive, intelligent, single thirty-two-year-old woman who has great difficulty maintaining a relationship, yet very much desires a husband and family. Although she is popular and easily gets dates, as soon as she feels emotionally close, she ends the relationship. For example, she will fail to show up at a meeting or appear inappropriately dressed for the occasion.

Her job history reflects the same pattern. She easily obtains employment, is well liked, and often rapidly advances to positions of greater responsibility, after which she will do something outlandish that ultimately leads to her dismissal. Her sudden changes baffle people, who conclude that she is an "odd duck."

Emma was raised in an affluent neighborhood, but her family had little money. Her father pursued get-rich-quick schemes that always failed, while her mother never spoke of the chronic financial insecurity the family suffered. Instead the mother kept expressing great enthusiasm for each of her husband's new ventures, believing that any current difficulties were surely transient and would soon be relieved. Told never to say anything of their plight to classmates or neighbors, the patient and her brother experienced themselves as valueless aliens who would be exposed as frauds at any moment.

The patient's brother also has difficulty sustaining relationships. However, he keeps a successful job—although he always anguishes that despite good performance, he will soon be seen as having no value and be fired. Emma reports that he often complains that the women he dates are good-looking but empty-headed. They are like putty to him; he can mold them as he wishes, but then he disrespects them as insubstantial.

It is easy to recognize the way Emma's parents created a false sense of identity for their family. Consequently, both children incorporated feelings of worthlessness into their Child states. As adults, both desire greater self-security and long to have their own families, but neither is able to fulfill what he or she desires in life. Emma's conduct in both her work and social life perpetuates her childhood identity as an impostor. This is certainly not what her Adult Wants, but it is what her Child Needs.

This powerful sense of worthlessness and insubstantiality *is* her identity, the paramount cue representing self, family, and home. In her work environment, she presents it as a calling card that says who she feels she is. Her actual skills and abilities dramatically contrast with this image. But maintaining success means losing her known identity. Holding on to her conflicted identity, however, will inevitably expose her as insubstantial. She fears loss either way.

Similarly, in social situations, Emma cannot allow herself to be close to a man lest her Child self be revealed. Consistent with the paradox of conflict, Emma tries to keep her negative self-perception in the dark by never talking about it, yet by her behavior she virtually advertises it in bright neon lights. *What is not talked out is acted out.* Emma paints herself into the very corner she so desperately tries to avoid by loudly broadcasting her dreaded, secret feelings through her behavior.

Lest you find yourself judgmental of her parents for creating such a plight for their children, keep in mind that there was never a parent who was not once a child. Instead we may reasonably ask: What unresolved conflicts from their own childhoods still haunt Emma's parents? How are these expressed in their familial relationships? What unresolved struggles did they inherit that are now being visited onto the next generation? It is not just Grandma's dishes to which subsequent generations become heirs.

Emma's mother grew up in a large, extended family. All of the members belonged to a fundamentalist religious group which believed that suffering in this life would be compensated for in the next, eternal life. She liked being different from her nonreligious peers in not being allowed to use makeup, dance, flirt, or date. She never expressed any resentment—at least not overtly. Nevertheless, she clearly acted out these feelings by choosing to marry Emma's father.

He was raised in a family in which the father was a charismatic, proudly atheistic, inveterate gambler, whom the son greatly admired. His mother complained constantly about her husband's irresponsibility and the family's financial instability. As an adult, Emma's father continued to express disgust for his mother's lack of support and constant criticism of her husband. "Pa would have done better if Ma had stopped the naggin'," he would say.

Now we can begin to see how the pieces fall into place. By choosing Emma's father, her mother was able to maintain her Child identity of long-suffering deprivation and differentness while covertly expressing her resentment by vicariously disowning any religious bonds. The patient's maternal grandparents were extremely upset by and opposed the mother's marriage. All the better! She could be in two places at the same time: complying with the familiarity of deprivation *and* rebelling against religion. Unfortunately both places spoke to the past, and neither expressed her Adult self.

Similarly, Emma's father's marriage to her mother enabled him to keep his Child identity with his own unrepentant father. Disliking his mother's nagging, he had chosen a woman who was antithetical to her. He convinced himself that he had a better marital relationship than his father had ever had—as though this ruse meant that he was superior to his own father. By choosing a wife who was an exact opposite of his mother, he tricked himself into imagining he had changed the familiar, only to end up in exactly the same situation—again, all **Child** and no **Adult**.

The relationship of Emma's parents demonstrates how when we consciously deny the existence of any conflict our minds have an amazing capacity to concentrate exactly on that which is emotionally important and to which we must attend. Consequently, slips of the tongue and behaviors inconsistent with intention speak volumes. A person's use of humor—the kinds of jokes he tells and the kinds he sees as funny—also provide a window into his mind. For this reason, patients in psychodynamic psychotherapy are encouraged to speak freely of whatever enters their minds, without censoring, even if the thought initially seems nonsensical. This is called *free association*. Dreams may be similarly understood—by simply going with the stream of thoughts that come to mind, like the pieces of a puzzle that, once assembled, create a picture not evident from any one piece alone.

Emma's unconscious struggle also illustrates how we focus on that which is emotionally most salient to us. Everyone calls her "Em." Her last name begins with a "T." She has chosen an e-mail address and license plate designation of "MT" without any conscious awareness of the profound message it conveys. She says that she wants a customized plate to avoid being "just ordinary." By her conduct, e-mail address, and license plate, she clearly advertises her worst, unacknowledged fear that she will be discovered to be "empty." The double entendre eludes her. *We always reveal what we try to conceal.*

I have oriented Emma's therapy to help her understand that she has condensed and incorporated her childhood experiences of feeling worthless into her patterns of behavior and even advertises this with her modified initials. Our focus on her extended family history has allowed Emma to recognize that she is not the only heir to valueless feelings. She came by these feelings honestly, so to speak, as did her parents, her brother, and relatives, whose life patterns she can now understand. Very likely, several former generations of her relatives have struggled similarly. Resolving the problem requires that she let go of her only emotionally known identity—MT—and acknowledge her *feeling* of emptiness by expressing the emotion verbally rather than behaviorally and from the perspective of being an **Adult**. Emma's journey of breaking free from what has kept her emotionally secure but imprisoned in her past—her Needs—will allow her a chance to have what she so much desires: her Wants.

Emma must take this step to reconcile her self-image with who she now is. She cannot eliminate her past, but by understanding, accepting, and integrating it, she can transcend the conflict. She has to know the Child but be the Adult. She has always Wanted to be healthy, of course, but her intense and powerful Need to hold onto her past identity, no matter how painful, lest she have none, has kept her chained to her childhood and to the trans-generational struggle for self-esteem. It may seem evident, but it is important to point out that if letting go of that dysfunctional identity had been easy to accomplish, she would have done it long ago.

When standing on the ledge of a burning building, it takes a person's leap of faith to hope the fireman's net will catch him if he jumps. *It is the Adult who holds the net for the adult person.* The therapist can support and encourage the patient taking "the chance on change" and may even do some preliminary catching, as when intervening to prevent a patient's suicide. But therapists can never be the ultimate catchers that the patient relies on. The patient's faith that he can let go of the past and move ahead is ultimately necessary.

Emma took the risk. She is able, slowly and tentatively, to unencumber herself through support; cognitive awareness of her considerable strengths; and encouragement to voice her feelings of sadness, grieve her childhood, and change the very behavior that has kept reinforcing her past identity. She fights against her tendency to negate her achievements and has gradually come to accept that her accomplishments are worthwhile—not just transient, valueless camouflage. She knows that she must constantly be on guard against falling back into the old familiar/familial patterns, but she feels confident about herself and her future. *The price of Adulthood is eternal vigilance. You must know where your Child is at all times.*

The Case of the Clothes Thief

Although not a patient of mine, a young woman whose case I describe next is another striking example of the remarkable way the mind constructs thoughts in an effort to balance the tensions of conflict. Jane was in her mid-twenties and volunteered to participate in a demonstration at a hypnosis conference. The therapist, Calvin Stein, who conducted a public portion of that program, introduced himself to her. He complimented Jane on her fashionable attire and attractive appearance. "Thank you," Jane said. "Everything I have on, including the handbag, the boots, and the belt, I've stolen." There was an expression of pride in her statement as audible as was the gasp from the audience. She went on to explain that she was a socialist, disgusted by the exploitation of the masses by heartless corporations driven by their lust for profits. Her stealing was a way of leveling the playing field just a little and making the corporations suffer for their avarice.

Jane, an excellent hypnotic subject, was soon in a deep trance. In this altered state of consciousness, Stein asked her to talk about her early childhood experiences. She described being the fourth daughter in a poor, hard-working family who could never afford to buy her new clothes. She always had to wear hand-me-downs from her three older sisters. She had internalized this perception, which formed her identity of never being entitled to anything new—her **Child's Need.** But she had also internalized healthy family values of right and wrong. The dilemma then became wanting new clothes, which she unconsciously perceived of as illegitimate, while maintaining the desire to be honest. Voilà! You can now appreciate her mental sleight of hand. She rationalized her behavior as a political statement that justified her stealing.

Jane's childhood experience became the essence of her emotional identity and created her sense of home and her place in the world—her Needs. Resolving the dilemma would have involved acknowledging her pain of deprivation as a child and grieving the loss of experiences she was entitled to have had but never did, such as wearing her own new clothes. This would have allowed her to be an **Adult** with legitimate Wants who could exercise real choice without the risk of being arrested. But because her Needs dictated her actions, she functioned as the Child masquerading as an adult. From her statements at the time, Jane clearly was not at all troubled by her behavior. Unless subsequently apprehended in her shoplifting activities or criticized by someone she cared about, it is unlikely that she would ever question her conduct, so powerful was her ability to rationalize.

Jane's story stuck in my mind as a vivid illustration of the enormous influence on the present person of her past identity as not being entitled to new clothing. It is also another demonstration of the mind's power to simultaneously reveal (by stealing) and conceal (by rationalizing) emotional conflict.

The Man who would Be Boss

George and Alice had been married for about eighteen years. Their relationship was clear and unambiguous. George was the unquestioned boss who micromanaged the household as well as his own successful business. As their children grew to greater independence, Alice, no longer satisfied with this long-standing status quo, gradually began to want a voice in matters that concerned their family—and so the trouble began.

Alice started by telling me about her overbearing mother, who never acknowledged anyone else's point of view. Her father was a quiet, reserved man who spent as much time as possible away from home, working in his moderately successful business. When he was at home, his conversations generally were limited to "Yes, dear." Alice abhorred her father's weakness as much as she detested her mother's dominance.

She saw her older brother and sister quietly gain more and more weight until both were obese as children and remained so as adults. Their weight was the one area of their lives over which Mother was constantly reminded that she had no control—as long as they remained fat. In other matters, her brother always deferred to the mother's dictates. He was unmarried but had had brief relationships, none of which the mother had found acceptable. The sister was married to a man who remained dependent on his family for advice and employment.

While growing up, Alice was popular, trim, athletic, and respected by her friends for her viewpoints. When she tried to bring that good feeling about herself and her opinions home, she ran into the brick wall of her mother's having to be in control. Not unlike Edvard Munch's famous painting *The Scream*, she felt that whatever she uttered was never heard, no matter how loudly she yelled. Although Alice could consciously voice her feelings of contempt for the family situation, she had internalized the pattern defining what constituted home, and that internalization formed her Child Needs.

Alice desperately wanted to be different from her mother. But from a child's point of view, mother is the most important female model, and Alice had an inner Need cue of her mother as the role model. As mentioned earlier, the Child can trick the adult into thinking that by doing the direct opposite of the Child's Needs, he is doing something different. In Alice's mind, as long as she did not speak up at home, she was not like her mother. But this left her just as she was as a child—unheard. Of course this was not what she desired.

She dated a number of nice young men who admired her intelligence, attractiveness, and points of view. Two of them proposed marriage, but they did not fit the map of what her Child Needed. Then along came George.

He grew up in a family that was the direct opposite of Alice's; his father was dominant and his mother submissive. His sister had married a man with whom she worked who was dominant just like George's father. However, unlike at home, in their business lives, the sister's husband did solicit her opinions and thoughts. She was much younger than George, so this probably represents a softening of the maturing parents' modeling. In addition, each sibling's differences of gender, personality, and experiences determined their varying adaptation to the same stimuli. For the sister and her husband, the work arena, unlike the home setting, may have been uncontaminated with the conflict of who should be in charge.

George's father's Need to control was so over-determined that it revealed what he needed to conceal and defend against: Feelings of inadequacy and insignificance. Alice's mother played the same power game. Their respective—but alas, *not respected*—spouses each overtly played the role of being the impotent, inadequate one. Both of the dominant parents had disowned their uncomfortable feelings of inferiority and projected them onto the spouses, who in turn accepted the projections, because the subservient role fit their familiar, unresolved Child Needs.

A teeter-totter symbolically represents the dominant-submissive relationship. The partner who is up and seems dominant actually depends for counterweight on the one who is down. Similarly, when a person says, "I choose you to be in charge of me," one may question who actually is in charge? Once more the paradox of conflict manifests itself. The overtly dominant one depends on the partner's submissive participation and is therefore equally dependent. Moreover, regardless of who is up and who is down, the distance between them remains the same and can change only if they decide to get off the teeter-totter.

George and Alice's dominant parents could become close with their spouses if they were willing to take back the impotent feelings they projected onto them. The submissive spouses had just as much power to change their situations. Making such a move, however, conjures up all the previously addressed fears of change—of going through zero. Rocking the boat might cause all to drown.

George had always taken control in his prior relationships. He dictated what was to be done and aggressively met anyone with a different point of view head-on. He acknowledged that this often caused the end of his relationships, as the women would not tolerate such dominance. Not realizing the significance of his behavior, he continued to dominate his partners, thinking that was just the way he was.

When George and Alice first met it was "love at first sight," unlike anything either had experienced in any previous relationship. They confused as love that powerful feeling of reconnecting with the familiarity that constituted "home." For both, their Child Need cues fit with those of the other. What a perfect match. Alice thought that she could not possibly be like her resented, dictatorial mother because George was reassuringly the one dictating. George could avoid confronting his feelings of insecurity because Alice, like his mother, was compliant. The balance was disrupted only with Alice's gradual maturation and growth. She was now more in touch with her desire to count in the relationship—or leave it.

George could give an intellectually affirmative nod to her wishes because he considered himself a modern man who respected a woman's equality. This was all well and good, except they never implemented the changes both said they desired. Instead they constantly argued and criticized each other, which finally brought them to therapy. On the surface, Alice seemed like the helpless victim of George's overbearing behavior. It would be tempting for a therapist to be drawn into siding with Alice against her bullying husband, but *what a mistake that would be*. The therapist must keep in mind and help the couple realize that their identical Child Needs drove them to collude in reestablishing the familiar/familial, a collusion antithetical to their Adult Wants.

Conflict in relationships, insofar as both people are participants, is a 50/50 proposition. Obviously each partner has 100 percent responsibility for his or her own contribution to the conflict. Alice's passivity played just as active a role as did George's dominance. Alice could fool herself into thinking that the problem was only George's opposition to her growth, because his behavior was so overtly constrictive. She could fancy the idea of solving this problem by leaving George if things did not work out. She thought of herself as attractive and was confident she would find a supportive partner if George would not change.

Clinical experience reveals that the Child's unsolved Needs will subsume the adult's desires when making the choice of a subsequent partner. This pattern certainly may be attenuated by maturity, but only if there is enough functioning Adult Want to overcome the Child Need. The history of remarriage—at least as evidenced by couples who come for therapy—indicates that people recapitulate their unexamined problems in the new unions. Therefore if Alice were to leave George at this stage, she would probably choose a partner psychologically similar to George with whom to work out her still unresolved childhood conflicts. Uninterrupted, the dance goes on.

Alice, in expressing her healthy desires, had not "owned" her Need for George to keep her in "protective custody." "The trouble with me is you," she pronounced. She had difficulty owning the 50 percent of the conflict her powerful passivity represented. To help identify those significant forces of emotional familiarity operating within her, I asked, "I know you don't Want George to behave the way he does, but why might you Need him to do so?" The question acknowledges and allies with her desire for change while simultaneously identifying her collusive role. Just as George could give verbal acknowledgment to valuing her as an equal partner, his Needs undercut her every tentative attempt to be one.

I emphasize again that Alice was not an innocent bystander in this dance but rather an active participant, maintaining what she Needed but did not Want, notwithstanding protestations to the contrary.

George and Alice illustrate that *every* adult relationship is composed of four points of reference: two **Adults** in real time and two **Child** selves representing past conflicts. It is the colluding "twinship" of their **Child** states that precipitates symptomatic behaviors. The intensity of that engagement depends on the residual power of their mutual struggles—their Needs. Partners act together to reestablish the shared essence of their homes of origin, whether desired or not. They emotionally rationalize that if the home they establish together thematically resembles the home of their childhoods, then they never have to leave home. If the residual conflicts are intense, resolving them—leaving home—feels like becoming orphaned.

Despite what is often said, it is not the couple's differences that generate their problems. Rather it is their sameness, the incredible synchronicity of the familiar/familial theme they share. This idea is more fully described in chapter five in the discussion of how we go about choosing mates. Although it is manifested differently—for him through domination, for her by acquiescence—both Alice and George suffer from profound feelings of insecurity. This powerful sameness, the tight-fitting familiar, is the intense attraction that is usually referred to as love at first sight. Less romantic perhaps, it more accurately should be called "familiarity at first sight."

I humorously caution people who are beginning or resuming dating to be wary of such immediate attraction. As wonderful as it may feel, it is likely fueled by the familiarity of themes from their early lives. If this is what they Want, and what they Need is resolved, the relationship can practically run on autopilot. If not, then they must work to break free of the past to be able to live in the present.

Because the compelling attraction formed by Needs is a given, the paramount issue is not the attraction per se. Rather each partner must recognize the unwanted patterns they both bring to their union and mutually commit to resolve, rather than perpetuate, those patterns.

I used the four stages of therapy described in Chapter Seven to help this couple disengage from their shared conflict. They identified the name of the game—George carried the onus of power, while Alice was saved from power's taint (being her mother)—and recognized the way they continued to play the game. I supported them in letting go of those patterns to allow the expression of their Adult desires. This third step of "quitting" the game represents letting go of the past—leaving the parental home—and embracing Adulthood.

Alice's passivity and George's aggression represented two sides of the same coin of their dilemma. Curiously enough, Alice found it more difficult than George to change her behavior. She had to face her intense fear of emotionally becoming like her mother if she expressed her thoughts and feelings. Until now, she had relied on George to save her from her fear of being destructive. The true alternative for Alice was to allow herself to appreciate that *being assertive is not synonymous with being aggressive*. As George disengaged from his defensive, controlling posture and felt more of an Adult himself, he became more receptive to Alice's Adult self. His surprising comfort with her speaking up was possible because he realized that he had previously unrecognized feelings of empathy for his mother's downtrodden plight.

The conflicted engagement of adults with one another is their own business—assuming the conduct is lawful and consensual—until they have children; then the stakes change. Too many parents busily raise patients for future therapists, passing their unresolved psychological issues on to the next generation. Alice and George, heirs to the unresolved problems of their own parents, were determined not to bequeath the same conflicts to their children.

The Bed as Battleground

Elliott and Martie thoroughly enjoyed their relationship prior to marriage. They had an active sexual relationship that was mutually satisfying. After living together for about three loving years, they decided to get married. That began a complete deterioration of their intimacy. They personified the popular expression that marriage can ruin a beautiful relationship. Elliott's sexual interest gradually declined during their first year of marriage, a source of great distress to Martie. Elliott complained that Martie now withheld the emotional support and encouragement he had enjoyed prior to marriage. They were locked in a vicious cycle: The less support Elliott received, the less he desired to be intimate; the less intimacy she received, the less support Martie felt like giving.

When I asked Martie about her family, she described being an only child and humorously wondered if she were immaculately conceived, since she knew from an early age that her parents did not have a sexual relationship. In fact, her mother expressed pride in not debasing herself with "animal" behavior. There was, however, no overt conflict between her parents—or much else. Her father was affable and well liked and enjoyed traveling. He kept busy with male friends. In contrast, Martie's mother stayed at home as much as possible, had few friends, and did not go on any trips with the father.

Martie recalled that her mother would always get very teary at the thought of her own father's death, which occurred when the mother was about ten years old. The grandfather had always been sickly and weak, and the grandmother had taken care of him as well as their two children while working to support the family. The grandmother never remarried. As a result Martie's mother incorporated an image of a wife as one who is burdened by a husband, a role model she did not wish to emulate. Although she married Martie's father, her life was quite separate from his, which fit his Need to avoid "settling down."

Martie, like her father, enjoyed traveling and keeping busy with friends. In her teens, she struggled with feelings of unattractiveness despite interest from boys who wanted to date her. Her first serious relationship was with a classmate in college. His never having any sexual interest in her intensified her concerns about her desirability and ultimately led her to end what she felt was an otherwise satisfactory relationship. Soon thereafter, she met Elliott through the aegis of her mother, who was an acquaintance of his mother's.

Elliott was the second of four children and the only boy. He described his mother as a "powerhouse who sweeps people along in her wake." The father was low-key and even-tempered and never complained about anything, seeming to take pride in his wife's considerable community influence and prominence. Elliott's older sister was obliged by the family to marry the man by whom she became pregnant at an early age. This marriage ended a few years later when it became known that the husband was physically abusive. The middle sister married a "jock" who was described as trying so hard to compensate for feelings of insecurity that he seemed a caricature. The youngest sister followed in the mother's footsteps, doing community work, and vowed never to marry. She was too satisfied with her life, she claimed, to ever sacrifice it for the sake of a husband.

Martie delighted in her new relationship, especially because Elliott showed great sexual enthusiasm and interest in her, expressing his good fortune to have such an attractive and exciting partner. And then they got married.

We are all symbolic creatures. Living together differs significantly from being married. It resembles playing house and does not become "real" until the rite of passage takes place. This is true whether a friend with a mail-order theology diploma officiates, the couple writes their own marriage vows, or they conduct the ceremony in the nude in a redwood forest. Once consecrated, the marriage becomes real, and old issues come to the fore. If the hidden agenda of emotionally powerful, unresolved Need emerges, it may deluge the couple's previously wonderful relationship.

Various important markers or rites of passage in addition to marriage may prompt the reemergence of unresolved conflicts. The birth of the first child, which signifies the birth of parenthood, may reawaken dormant issues around parental roles. Other examples could be the year reached in the marriage that coincides with when parents divorced; the birth of a child who symbolically recapitulates sibling issues; reaching the same age at which a parent died; or any internalized remarkable childhood event emotionally attached to a date and time. Any significant symbolic event may trigger the expression of unexplored Needs. Such is the power of symbolism.

For Martie and Elliott it was their marriage that brought forth their insecurities. Martie began to question her value as a woman, particularly her sexual role. Although convinced that Elliott was nothing like her prior boyfriend and that their marriage differed completely from that of her parents, lo and behold, she was "back home" again. Elliott expressed insecurities about his role as a man, which had been kept at bay so well by Martie's continued reassurances during their courtship, by withdrawing into a secondary role. He felt "neutered," just as he perceived his father had been by his overbearing mother.

When I asked about Elliott's sisters and their relationships, it became evident that they were all "marinated" in the familial theme of the insignificant man and the strong woman. Two sisters chose men who suffered from their own severe insecurities. The abusive husband acted out his disowned feelings of denigration; for the same reason, the jock husband behaved like a cartoon character, which only invited people to disregard him. Although the sisters chose men seemingly unlike their father, each ended up "back home" as the dominant woman with a weak man. The third sister, modeling herself directly after the mother, dismissed men as irrelevant, rationalizing that her community work left her no time for a relationship. She never even bothered to try to leave home, symbolically or literally. Each of the sisters either directly or indirectly took different "roads to Rome." But they all ended up sacrificing their Wants to satisfy their Needs.

Martie and Elliott's therapy focused on their understanding of how and why they danced to the despised old familiar melodies—the powerful woman and insignificant man. They recognized that they required help to get away from this conflicted paradox. Their behavior after marriage, neither capricious nor random, represented precisely what they feared most as adults—being themselves seen as they saw their parents: inadequate or dominating (two sides of the same coin). They had defended against those painful feelings by denying them, thereby entrenching themselves in perpetuating the very behaviors that fed the cycle of feeling deficient. They had painted themselves into the corner they wanted to avoid and were highly motivated to change.

As they began to comprehend the message their behavior conveyed and gave voice to their childhood feelings, they appreciated the similarity of their struggles and the reason they were drawn to each other. Martie and Elliott wanted a marriage in which they were equal partners, each valuing and respecting the other. However, they lacked the emotional precedent from their families of origin on which to call and had to blaze their own trail. By increasingly expressing mutual appreciation, they reclaimed what they valued about their early years together. The initial strength of that time provided a foundation for building a stable structure that could withstand those stressful times when one or the other would regress to old postures. Their understanding of how the forces of their **Child Needs** pitted against their **Adult Wants** along with their increased empathy with their parents and siblings buttressed that foundation.

Since their marriage they had gradually alienated themselves from their families of origin, perhaps subliminally recognizing that their problems grew out of their early family life experiences. By understanding their families' emotional struggles, expressed—paradoxically—through perpetuating adverse behaviors, they reversed this withdrawal and began a growth process that could form the basis for a healthy life together. Facing the fearful feelings of inadequacy that had confined them to the past allowed them to feel confident that they are good enough both as individuals and as a couple.

Sexual Symptoms

I want to refer back to Martie and Elliott's complaint about their relationship's lack of sex. Sexual symptoms—whether the initial presenting complaint or collateral damage from other problems—may be divided into two categories: Physiological and psychological.

Physiological sexual problems have medical causes for which there are effective medical treatments. For example, physical abnormalities, medications, and medical conditions such as diabetes or low testosterone or estrogen levels may interfere with sexual performance. In such cases a variety of medical treatments can establish or restore healthier sexual functioning.

The psychological sexual symptoms, in turn, can be divided into two subcategories: Those stemming from *ignorance* and those caused by *displacement*. Sexual ignorance pervades American culture. Somehow our society deems it advisable to have peers or senior peers (kids a few years older) conduct sexual education furtively and in incongruous places. Those "professors" usually have access to explicit materials or, putatively, have had some sexual experiences themselves. I applaud those parents who recognize their children's curiosity and in an ongoing, age-appropriate fashion give them intelligent information about sex. Such parents are unusual, however, and so a great deal of either complete ignorance or abysmal misinformation regarding sex abounds in our society among both youths and older people.

Directly providing sexual information, clarification, and education may eliminate ignorance-generated conflict in the bedroom. Sometimes simply letting patients give voice to their interests, fantasies, and wishes and assuring them of their normalcy suffices, thereby eliminating the need to employ specific sex therapy techniques.

Sexual symptoms caused by displacement have nothing to do with sex at all. On the contrary, other problems acted out in the sexual arena take the form of sexual difficulties, which Martie and Elliott's relationship illustrates. They initially enjoyed a healthy and satisfying adult sexual relationship. Only after they married did their healthy sex life get usurped to express their shared unresolved Child conflicts, presented as though those conflicts were sexual.

Utilizing sex therapy techniques without determining what the symptoms mean may miss the whole "message in the medium" and not resolve the problems. A well-constructed dynamic formulation is essential in such cases. If a couple can override the conflicts with structured exercises aimed at resuming intimate contact, behavioral techniques may prove successful. If not, they must attend to the underlying issues, which masquerade as sexual difficulties.

The Husband Who Wasn't

Joe came to therapy complaining of physical and emotional exhaustion. He had been obliged throughout his entire childless, thirty-five year marriage to maintain two full-time jobs to satisfy his wife's financial demands. Having never complained before, he found bearing the burden more difficult as he aged. In light of his description, it astounded me to hear that each and every month his wife, Jan, received a substantial amount of interest money from a very large trust.

Joe described having been raised in the shadow of his cousin—a world-famous person whom he physically resembled. In fact, people frequently mistook him for the cousin because of the striking similarity in their appearances and then dropped him like a hot potato after realizing their mistake. Conversations with social acquaintances or work associates seemed continually to center upon their desire for information about his cousin's life, family, interests, and current activities.

After several sessions it became evident that Joe desperately wanted his wife to know how much he struggled with financial burdens, but he had no idea how to approach her. I suggested that he ask her to come to an interview session with him. I specifically chose the term *interview* and not *therapy* so that she would feel more comfortable with the invitation. This is a useful way of having significant others participate without fearing that they have to commit to therapy themselves.

Joe had described his feeble attempts over the years to discuss the household finances with his wife, which had only resulted in her becoming dismissive and annoyed, telling him not to bother her with such meaningless matters. The finances were his responsibility, she had told him. Certainly such petty matters never bothered her father.

Jan entered the consultation room looking like an aging southern belle with a flounced skirt and large, floppy-brimmed hat. She had the air of a perpetual teenager about her, in sharp contrast to her slightly built, stooped, aged-beyond-his-years husband. She said that she was curious about me and puzzled why her husband was making such a fuss. She described her family by focusing on her long-deceased, self-made multimillionaire father, whom she idealized. She spoke of him in glowing, elaborate, hyperbolic terms. He was larger than life. No man she had ever met approached his level of achievement and perfection. She pointedly made this statement at our first meeting and with her husband—more like a fixture than a person in her presence—sitting next to her.

Her continued effusive portrayal of her father soon revealed, between the lines, a chauvinistic misogynist. Without any awareness, she outlined conduct demonstrating her father's contempt for women, including her mother and herself. Her father had invested all of his trust and positive expectations in her brother while ignoring the brother's continued failures; instead he heaped encouragement on his son to keep on trying, even as he undercut the son's efforts in business. To say that she was unconsciously ambivalent about her father would be a vast understatement.

The father's dismissal of women as being fit only for the kitchen and the nursery probably influenced his decision to establish his trust fund so that his daughter could draw only on the interest each month. Nonetheless, this amounted to a sizable sum. After Jan's death, the principle would go to her brother and his children, as well as certain specified organizations of interest to the father. There was no mention of her husband.

Despite Joe's (albeit inept) pleas for her financial assistance, Jan declined and continued every month to purchase all kinds of clothing, shoes, jewelry, accessories, makeup, and so on, dissipating the entire monthly sum. She dismissed her husband's requests for help by reiterating that it was his duty to be the financial provider. She had incorporated the image of herself from the family model of an empty-headed, superficial, irresponsible woman who could not be trusted with money matters. While busily expressing her overt contempt for her husband's plight, she covertly revealed her utter disdain for her father and his money by her shopping behavior, paradoxically validating her father's view of women.

This couple's twinship collusion of **Child Needs** clearly meshed and kept them together. Jan complied with the view of herself as having little substance while extolling her great father's virtues. Emotionally locked in the past, she longed for her father's acknowledgment and approval while perpetually engaging in behaviors that he would have abhorred. Joe continued to live in a great man's shadow, never feeling that he was a valued person in his own right and wishing that at least his wife would recognize his worth.

I wish I could report that Joe and Jan progressed toward a satisfactory resolution of their mutual conflict, able to experience themselves and each other more as Adults enjoying what they Wanted. However, that is not the case. At a subsequent session I ever so gently suggested that perhaps, as with all real people, Jan's father might have had some emotional issues himself. Jan abruptly stood up, demanded an apology, and stalked out of the office. All subsequent attempts to contact her to discuss what had happened were of no avail. Joe continued therapy for a few more sessions. He intellectually acknowledged and understood the meaning of what had transpired and how much *both* his and Jan's behaviors made sense in light of the *mutual* synergistic forces brought forward from their childhoods.

Because of his wife's refusal to reflect on her behavior, Joe realized that their relationship probably would not change much. However, he found the situation easier to live with, he said, now that he understood the emotional meaning of their behaviors. Recognizing his greater personal significance felt both satisfying and dangerous, as it meant facing frightening consequences if he were to be too assertive and break away from his accustomed second-class role. As much as he felt victimized, Joe now knew that the conflict was not just of Jan's making. He concluded the therapy with expressions of appreciation for having been heard and understood. Though this was a rather modest achievement compared with what might have been possible, it was certainly worthwhile and as far as Joe dared go. Considering his assertion that he had never before in his entire life felt listened to or heard, it was a monumental experience.

Earlier I used the metaphor of the Hebrew slaves leaving the security of Egyptian bondage only to face the zero of the desert. Referring to that image, I do not believe Joe would have allowed himself to go very far beyond the city limits. Nevertheless, in the metaphor of the Calder mobile lies some optimism and hope for this couple. The movable sculpture illustrates the fact that when any one piece of the system changes, so does the entire system's balance. In this case, Joe's understanding led to his standing and walking straighter, as actually seen in his posture when he left therapy, in contrast to when he started. Predictably, this very subtle change could have an ultimate effect on their relationship and on Jan's attitude toward him. This phenomenon, though of unknown impact on Joe and Jan, has been seen in many situations in which one person's modest gain in a relationship or family magnifies over time and influences the other(s) to change as well. It is the "butterfly effect" to which I referred in discussing chaos theory.

Another metaphor might be helpful in recognizing the value of small changes. Even if a sailor alters his course by a negligible compass degree, the ship will arrive in an entirely different port than previously expected. Therefore, therapists should remember that small changes can lead to large ones and not be discouraged when their diligent work seems to be for naught. Perhaps the poignant title of Milton Erickson's book *My Voice Will Go with You*[6] can serve as a reminder.

Before the days of television, there was a weekly radio program called *Grand Central Station,* which dramatized stories of people in New York City. Each broadcast had an introductory statement that said, "Grand Central Station! Crossroads of a million private lives! Gigantic stage on which are played a thousand dramas daily!" The program provided an opportunity to understand the struggles of individuals, couples, and families and the emotional similarities of all human beings. The clinical examples discussed here have the same purpose: To illustrate the powerful hold that our past perceptions have on our present lives as well as the difficulty of letting go of those perceptions, the feelings they induce, and the consequent behavior that may run counter to what we desire. In other words, how difficult it is to break free of the once Needed childhood chains that kept us safe but now keep us from what we Want.

CHAPTER TEN

Synopsis

We hope that the ideas we have presented in this book will help make emotional conflict more understandable and explain why changing symptomatic behavior poses such a challenge. If our adult desires differ from what we learned to need as children, it beckons from the other side of a void. Reaching what we yearn for requires a willingness to give up the learned perceptions that have given us a sense of security and predictability but keep us from attaining our desired goals by chaining us to the past. To break free from the chains that bind us to the past, we must face the void of letting go of the old while not yet having the new. The profundity of the void varies in depth and breadth with each individual—depending on the quality of the nature (biological factors) and nurturing each has received. The greater our confidence in taking sensible risks, the easier it is for us to replace old with new experiences, and the shallower and narrower the void seems.

The terms **Child** and **Adult**, modified from those introduced by Berne, usefully separate states of being that are parts of all of us to varying proportions. Disturbing feelings and symptomatic behaviors result from the clash between the two forces of **Adult Wants** and **Child Needs**.

In our thesis we have emphasized that as young children we learn how to behave and what conditions we need to survive. These are the learned cues, or prototypes, that form our **Child Needs**. The power imbued in this learning derives from the unique circumstances inherent in childhood. In our earliest state of helpless dependence, no alternatives exist to whatever our caretaking situation is—other than loss of survival. Because we have no options, we idealize those cues that define our existence and internalize this idealization in the form of familiar/familial patterns that ultimately serve to ensure our emotional survival through sameness. This represents our **Child**—manifested by the Need to maintain those cues that gave us a sense of self, others, and the world. Desperately staying in the known, then-and-there stance of the past, we dispel uncertainty and maintain predictability—even if we do not want the outcome and intellectually understand it to be painful or destructive.

In contrast, as we mature and begin to develop an **Adult** self, we become increasingly capable of expressing what we Want in the here and now. When the **Adult** Wants are the same as the **Child** Needs, little conflict ensues, because we incorporate those Needs into our Wants. Very few people are so blessed. More commonly, a state of tension exists between these two forces. Our **Child** self, imbued with powerful emotions associated with survival, tries to combat change, and our **Adult** self can easily be sidelined by this intense effort for continuity. The confronting interface between here-and-now **Adult** Wants and then-and-there **Child** Needs defines our struggle to grow as individuals, couples, families, and communities.

When as children we have sufficient support from our significant others to risk questioning the status quo and make changes, it becomes far easier for us as adults to tolerate *both* the unfamiliar on the one hand and the loss of the familiar on the other. We stress *both* in that each has its own emotional dimensions. Letting go of the *known* pain of deleterious behaviors and facing the fear of the *unknown* that change brings are both crucial factors in growth and essential tasks to complete before we can strike our chains and go through zero—the void—on the way to our desired goals.

Successfully rearing a child means giving that emerging self the confidence that he can handle whatever comes along in his life in the best way possible and that he will learn from and grow with his experiences as long as his efforts are viewed as self-enhancing and mistakes are seen as opportunities to improve.

Relinquishing whatever we once perceived to be vital, familiar, and predictable but that now blocks our ability to achieve greater fulfillment is a profound and difficult step. Watch children play the game *Touch Home and You Are Safe*. The rules say you cannot be tagged out if you touch the safe object called "home." But at the same time you cannot reach the winning goal, which may be some distance away, without letting go of the safe. A child desperately stretches to reach that goal while simultaneously holding onto the safety of home. He cannot succeed unless the goals are extremely limited—or the venture entirely forfeited. It is equally impossible to reach what we Want as **Adults** while still holding onto our **Child** Needs. The void (zero) must be traversed.

Our wish for you is: *Know what you Need, but have what you Want; Love the Child, but be the Adult.*

REFERENCES

Citations labeled as personal communication refer to comments made at large meetings, small group gatherings, or specifically to me and took place over a wide span of time, making it impossible to cite exact places and dates. My intention is to give credit for the comments made.

Introduction

1. Ridley, M. (2003). *Nature via Nurture.* New York: Harper Collins.
2. Steinberg, D. (2006). Determining nature vs. nurture. *Scientific American Mind,* October–November.
3. Gallagher, W. (1994). How we become what we are. *Atlantic Monthly,* September.
4. Brownlee, C. (2005). Twins' gene regulation isn't identical. *Science News,* July 9.
5. Your brain and psychotherapy. (2006). *Harvard Mental Health Letter* 23 (August).
6. The neurobiology of psychotherapy. (2006). *Psychiatric Annals* 36 (April).
7. Brunon, J., Kardener, S., and Karno, M. (1975). *Generative Graphics: Image Making in Psychotherapy.* Los Angeles: Behavioral Science Media Lab, University of California. Film presented at the American Psychiatric Association Annual Meeting.

Chapter 1

1. Seligman, M. (2002). *Helplessness.* New York: W. H. Freeman.
2. Masterson, J. F. (2000). *The Personality Disorders.* Phoenix: Zeig Tucker.
3. Functional brain imaging. (1998). *Primary Psychiatry,* March.

Neuroimaging finds biological basis of disorders. (1999). *Clinical Psychiatry News,* February.

4. Greenberg, J. R., and Mitchell, S. A. (1983). *Object Relations in Psychoanalytic Theory.* Cambridge, MA: Harvard University Press. Hamilton, G. N. (1989). A critical review of object relations theory. *American Journal of Psychiatry* 146 (December).

5. Anderson, S. W., Bechara, A., Damasio, H., et al. (1999). Impairment of social and moral behavior related to early damage in human prefrontal cortex. *Nature Neuroscience* 2 (November).

6. Kardener, S. H. (1968). The family: Structure, patterns, and therapy. *Mental Hygiene* 52 (October).

7. Fairbairn, W. R. D. (1954). *An Object Relations Theory of the Personality.* New York: Basic Books. Freud, S. (1958). Mourning and melancholia. *Standard Edition of the Complete Psychological Works of Sigmund Freud.* London: Hogarth Press.

8. Dietrich, D. J. (1976). Dietrich Tiedemann: Child psychologist of the 18th century. *Historian* 38.

9. Darwin, C. (1877). Biographical sketch of an infant. *Mind* 2.

10. Binet, A. (1903). *Etude Experimentale de L'intelligence.* Paris: Schleicher.

11. Piaget, J. (1955). *The Language and Thought of the Child.* New Haven, CT: Meridian Books, Noonday Press.

12. Stern, D. N. (1985). *The Interpersonal World of the Infant: A View from Psychoanalytic and Developmental Psychology.* New York: Basic Books. Stern, D. N. (1977). *The First Relationships: Mother and Infant.* Cambridge, MA: Harvard University Press. Ainsworth, M. D. S., et al. (1978) *Patterns of Attachment: A Psychological Study of the Strange Situation.* Mahwah, NJ: Erlbaum.

13. Father's role (2005). Ohio State University Extension Fact Sheet. Family and Consumer Sciences.

14. *Ibid.*

15. Lynn, D. B. (1974). *The Father: His Role in Child Development.* Belmont, CA: Wadsworth. Rohner, R., and Veneziano, R. (2001). The importance of father love: History and contemporary evidence. *Review of General Psychology,* December.

16. *Ibid.*

17. Johnson, J. G. (2006). Parenting behaviors associated with risk for the personality disorders during adulthood. *Archives of General Psychiatry* 63 (May).

18. Kohut, H. (1977). *Restoration of the Self.* New York: International Universities Press.
19. Shore, A. N. (1994). *Affect Regulation and the Origins of the Self.* Mahwah, NJ: Erlbaum.
20. Farb, P. (1978). *Humankind.* Boston: Houghton Mifflin.
21. Spitz, R. (1945). Hospitalism: An inquiry into the genesis of psychiatric conditions in early childhood. *Psychounalytic Study of the Child* 1.
22. Carlson, M., and Earls, F. (1997). Psychological and neuroendocrinological sequelae of early social deprivation in institutionalized children in Romania. *Annals of the New York Academy of Science* 807.
23. Nelson, C.A., and Bloom, F. E. (1997). Child development and neuroscience. *Child Development* 68.
24. Harlow, H. F. (1958). The nature of love. *American Psychologist* 123.
25. Winnicott, D. W. (1953). Translational objects and transitional phenomena. *International Journal Psychoanalysis* 34. Fromm, G. M., and Smith, B. L. (eds). (1989). *The Facilitating Environment: Clinical Applications of Winnicott's Theory.* Madison, CT: International Universities Press.
26. Masterson, *Personality Disorders.*
27. Winnicott, D. W. (1965). *The Maturational Processes and the Facilliatating Enviornment.* New York: International Universities Press.
28. Shore, A. N. (1998). Understanding and treating trauma: Developmental and neurobiological approaches. University of California at Los Angeles, Continuing Education Seminar.
29. Shore, A. N. (1997). Early organization of the nonlinear right brain and development of a predisposition to psychiatric disorders. *Development and Psychopathology* 5 (Fall).
30. Alexander's corrective emotional experience. (1997) in *Great Ideas in Psychotherapy* (Chessick, R. ed.). New York: Aronson.
31. Masterson, *Personality Disorders.*
32. Shore, Early organization of the nonlinear right brain.
1. Siegel, D. J. (1999). *The Developing Mind: Toward a Neurobiology of Interpersonal Experience.* New York: Guilford.
33. Ainsworth et al., *Patterns of Attachment.*
34. Siegel, *The Developing Mind.*

35. Weinberger, D. R. (1999). Neurogenesis occurs throughout the lifespan. *Clinical Psychiatry News,* March.

36. Hubel, D. H., and Wiesel, T. N. (1962). Receptive fields, binocular interaction and functional architecture in the cat's visual cortex. *Journal of Physiology* 160.

37. Ostrovsky, Y., Andalman, A., and Sinha, P. (2006). Vision following extended visual blindness. *Psychological Science* 17 (December).

38. Cicchetti, D. (2004). An odyssey of discovery: Lessons learned through three decades of research on child maltreatment. *American Psychologist* 59 (November).

39. Main, M. (1996). Introduction to the special section on attachment and psychopathology: 2. Overview of the field of attachment. *Journal of Counseling and Clinical Psychology* 64.

40. Chiron, C., Jambaque, I., Nabbout, R., et al. (1997). The right brain is dominant in human infants. *Brain* 120.

41. Gazzaniga, M. S. (1998). Split brain revisited. *Scientific American,* July.

42. Gillespie, C. F., and Nemeroff, C. B. (2005). Early life stresses and depression. *Current Psychiatry* 4 (December).

43. Grotstein, J. S. (1990). Nothingness, meaninglessness, chaos, and the "black hole." *Contemporary Psychoanalysis* 26.

44. Thousands Hear Dalia Lama's Message during Emory U. ceremony, http://www.pbs.org/weta/washigntonweek/voices/200710/1022world0.

45. Bowlby, J. (1949). *The Making and Breaking of Affectional Bonds.* New York: Tavistock Publications.

46. Ainsworth et al., *Patterns of Attachment.*

2. Karen, R. (1990). Becoming attached. *Atlantic Monthly,* February.

47. Kummer, J., personal communication.

48. Miller, M. (ed.). (2005). The biology of child maltreatment: How abuse and neglect of children leave their mark on the brain. *Harvard Mental Health Letter* 21 (June).

49. Miller, M. (ed.). (2004). The sadness and pain of rejection. *Harvard Mental Health Letter* 20 (June).

50. Kluger, J. (2005). The paradox of supermax. *Time,* February 5.

51. Nash, J. M. (1997). Fertile minds. Special report. *Time,* February 3.

52. Siegel, D. (1998). Understanding and treating trauma:

Developmental and neurobiological approaches. University of California, Los Angeles, Continuing Education Seminar.
53. Gladwell, M. (2005). *Blink: The Power of Thinking without Thinking.* New York: Little, Brown.
54. Mehrabian, A. (1971). *Silent Messages.* Belmont, CA: Wadsworth.
55. McLuhan, M. H., Fiore, Q., and Agel, J. (1967). *The Medium is the Massage: An Inventory of Effects.* New York: Bantam Books.
56. Sandifor, J. R., Hordern, A., and Green, L. M. (1970). The psychiatric interview: The impact of the first three minutes. *American Journal of Psychiatry* 126 (January).
57. Carrere, S., and Gottman, J. M. (1999). Predicting divorce among newlyweds from the first three minutes of a marital conflict discussion. *Family Process* 38.
58. Siegel, Understanding and treating trauma.
59. Siegel, *The Developing Mind.*
60. *Ibid.*

Chapter 2

1. Berne, E. (1986). *Transactional Analysis in Psychotherapy.* (reissued ed.). New York: Ballantine Books.
2. Piaget, J. (1926). *Judgment and Reasoning in the Child.* New York: Harcourt. Lin, S. (2002) Piaget's developmental stages. In *Encyclopedia of Educational Technology,* Hoffman, B. (ed.). San Diego State University, San Diego, CA.
3. *Little Oxford Dictionary of Quotations.* (2005). New York: Oxford University Press. This is one of several versions attributed to St. Ignatius of Loyola and quoted in the British House of Parliament debates, January 21, 2004 and October 31, 2006.
4. Kuhn, D., Langer, J., Kohlberg, L., and Haan, N. S. (1977). The development of formal operations in logical and moral judgements. *Genetic Psychology Monographs* 95.
5. Fairbairn, *An Object Relations Theory of the Personality.*
6. May, R. (1969). *Love and Will.* New York: W. W. Norton.
7. Ramen, R. N., personal communication.
8. Solzhenitsyn, A. I. (2002). *The Gulag Archipelago.* New York: Harper Collins.
9. Freud, S. (1958). The ego and the id. *Standard Edition of the Complete Works of Sigmund Freud.* London: Hogarth Press.

10. Milton, J. (1608-1674). *Paradise Lost. A Poem in 10 Books.* http://gutenburg.org/etext/26

11. Epictetus, Greek philosopher. (55-135 CE.) *The Golden Sayings of Epictetus.* http://www.gutenberg.org/etext/871

12. Frankl, V. E. (1959) *Man's Search for Meaning: An Introduction to Logotherapy.* Boston: Beacon Press.

Chapter 3

1. Berne, E., (1947). *The Mind in Action.* New York: Simon and Schuster.

2. West, L. J. (1985) On prejudice. *Grand Rounds.* Los Angeles: University of California, Neuropsychiatric Institute.

3. West, L. J. (1967). The psychobiology of racial violence. *Archives of General Psychiatry* 16 (June).

4. Gup, T. (2004). Tolerance has never come naturally (editorial). *Washington Post*, March 14.

5. Coined by Nils Bejerot, MD. (1973). Swedish radio broadcast, August 28.

1. Graham, D. L., and Rawlings, E. L. (1991) Bonding with abusive dating partners: Dynamics of the Stockholm syndrome. In *Dating Violence: Women in Danger* (Levy, B ed.). Seattle: New Leaf (Seal Press).

6. *Kitzmiller, et.al. v. Dover Area School District, et.al.* (2005). Judge John E. Jones. U.S. District Court Case No. 04cv2688, December 20.

7. Proust, M. (1925). *The Sweet Cheat Gone* (Vol. 2). New York: Random House.

8. Ramen, R. N., personal communication.

9. Freud, S. (1958). Project for a scientific psychology. *Standard Edition of the Complete Psychological Works of Sigmund Freud.* London: Hogarth Press.

10. Grotjahn, M., personal communication.

11. Grotstein, J., personal communication.

12. Grotjahn, M. personal communication.

13. McNamara, R. (1995). *In Retrospect: The Tragedy and Lessons of Vietnam.* New York: Times Books.

14. Santayana, G. (1905). *The Life of Reason* (Vol. 1). New York: Scribner and Sons.

15. Medawar, J., and Pyke, D. (2001). *Hitler's Gift. The True Story*

of the Scientists Expelled by the Nazi Regime. New York: Arcade Publishing.

16. Jack Smith, (1958-1996). *Los Angeles Times* columnist.

17. Oxford English Dictionary. (1987). Compact edition. Oxford: Oxford University Press.

18. Griffin, S. F. (ed.). (1990). *The Autobiograpy of William Allen White* (2nd ed.). Lawrence, KS: University Press of Kansas.

Chapter 4

1. Rainey, A. (2008). Shasu or Habiru: Who were the Early Israelites? *Biblical Archaeology Review* 34 (November/December).

2. Rabkin, R. (1968). Is the unconscious necessary? *American Journal of Psychiatry* 125 (September).

3. Fine, R. (1973) *The Development of Freud's Thoughts.* New York: Aronson.

4. James, W. (1902). *The Varieties of Religious Experience.* New York: Viking-Penguin, Reprinted 1982.

5. Fromm, E. (1959). Sigmund Freud's mission: An analysis of his personality and influence. In *World Perspectives* (vol. 21). New York: Harper.

6. Akenside, M. (1744). *Pleasures of the Imagination.* Bk.1, 1.23. in Stevenson, B. (ed.). (1965). Macmillan Book of Proverbs, Maxims, and Famous Phrases. New York. Macmillan.

7. Berne, E. (1964). *Games People Play: The Psychology of Human Relationships.* New York: Grove Press.

8. Berne, E. (1969). Demonstration interview of a family. Los Angeles: University of California, Neuropsychiatric Institute.

9. Grotstein, J., personal communication.

10. Jackson, D. (1965). Family rules: Marital quid pro quo. *Archives of General Psychiatry* 12.

11. Greenson, R., personal communication.

12. O'Donohoe, B. (2005). Why Sartre matters. *Philosophy Now* 53.

13. Bowen, M. (1985) *Family Therapy in Clinical Practice.* New York. Aronson.

14. Yalom, I., personal communication.

Chapter 5

1. Buss, D. M. (1994) *The Evolution of Desire: Strategies of Human Mating.* New York: Basic Books.

2. Diamond, J. (1998). Survival of the sexiest. *Discover*, May.
3. Bertman, S. (2008). Love at first sight. *Skeptical Inquirer* 32 (November/December).
4. Kardener, S. H. (1970). Convergent internal security systems: A rationale for marital therapy. *Family Process* 9 (March).
5. Stoller, R., personal communication.
6. Bowen, M. (1985). *Family Therapy in Clinical Practice*. New York. Aronson.
7. Witaker, C., personal communication.
8. Hertz, J. H. (1945) *Sayings of the Fathers*. New York: Behrman House.
9. Feiffer cartoon. (1974). *Field Newspaper Syndicate:* 9–8.
10. Masterson, J. F. (1976). *Psychotherapy of the Borderline Adult: A Developmental Approach*. New York: Bruner Mazel.
11. Eco, U. (1998). *Serendipities: Language and Lunacy*. New York: Columbia University Press.
12. Minuchin, S., personal communication.
13. Dawkins, R. (1990). *The Selfish Gene*. New York: Oxford University Press.

Chapter 6

1. Alexander, F. G., and Selesnick, S. T. (1966). *The History of Psychiatry*. New York: Harper & Row.
2. Kaufman, W. (1970). *I and Thou: Martin Buber*. New York: Scribners.
3. Greenson, R. (1967). *Technique and Practice of Psychoanalysis*. Madison, CT. International Universities Press.
4. Berne, E. (1966). *Principles of Group Treatment*. New York: Oxford University Press.
5. Jones, E. (1961). *The Life and Work of Sigmund Freud*. New York: Basic Books.
6. Viorst, J. (1986) *Necessary Losses*. New York: Simon and Schuster.
7. Ramen, R. N., personal communication.
8. Stoller, R. (1968). *Sex and Gender: On the Development of Masculinity and Femininity*. Santa Rosa, CA: Science House.
9. Perry, S., et al. (1987). The psychodynamic formulation: Its purpose, structure, and clinical application. *American Journal of Psychiatry* 144 (May). Ross, C.A., et al. (1990). Psychiatric case

formulation: A method of teaching and evaluating. *Academic Psychiatry* 14 (Summer).

10. McMullin, R. E. (2000). *The New Handbook of Cognitive Therapy Techniques.* New York: W. W. Norton. DeRubeis, R. J., and Beck, A. T. (1988). Cognitive therapy. In *Handbook of Cognitive-Behavioral Therapies.* (Dobson, K. S., ed.). New York: Guilford.

11. Freud, S. (1958). Remembering, repeating, and working through. In *Standard Edition of the Complete Psychological Works of Sigmund Freud.* London: Hogarth Press.

12. Masterson, J. F. (1981). *The Narcissistic and Borderline Disorders: An Integrated Developmental Approach.* New York: Bruner Mazel.

13. Perls, F. (1971). *Gestalt Therapy Verbatim.* New York: Bantam Books.

14. http://bipolar.about.com/cs/humor/a/00082_smile.htm   http://longevity.about.com/od/lifelongbeauty/tp/smiling.htm

Chapter 7

1. Kardener, S. H. (1975). A methodological approach to crisis therapy. *American Journal of Psychotherapy* 29 (January).

2. Parad, H. J. (ed.). (1965). *Crisis intervention: Selected readings.* New York: Family Services Association.

3. Ursano, R. J., and Hales, R. E. (1986). A review of brief individual therapies. *American Journal of Psychiatry* 143 (December).

4. Klerman, G. L. (1968). The psychiatric patient's right to effective treatment: Implications of Osheroff v. Chestnut Lodge. *American Journal of Psychiatry* 147.

5. Mandel, A. (1967). Psychoanalysis and psychopharmacology. In *Modern Psychoanalysis: New Directions and Perspectives* (Marmor, J., ed.). New York: Basic Books. Uhlenhuth, E. H., et al. (1969). Combined pharmacotherapy and psychotherapy. *Journal of Nervous and Mental Disease* 148. Group for the Advancement of Psychiatry Report. (1975). *Pharmacotherapy and Psychotherapy: Paradoxes, Problems, and Progress.* Arlington, MD: Mental Health Materials Center.

6. Kramer, P. (1993). *Listening to Prozac.* New York: Penguin Books.

7. Wright, J. H., and Hollifield, M. (eds.). (2006). Combining pharmacotherapy and psychotherapy. *Psychiatric Annals* 36 (May).

8. Wohlberg, L. R. (1972). *Hypnosis: Is it for You?* New York: Harcourt, Brace Jovanovich.
9. Orne, M. T., Sheehan, P. W., and Evans, F. J. (1968). Occurrence of posthypnotic behavior outside the experimental setting. *Journal of Personality and Social Psychology*
10. Orne, M. T., personal communication.
11. O'Donohue, W., and Krasner, L. (1997). *Theories of Behavioral Change.* Arlington, MD: APA Press. Dobson, K. S. (1988). *Handbook of Cognitive-Behavioral Therapies.* New York: Guildford Press.
12. Gordon, T. (1970). *Parent Effectiveness Training: The Proven Program for Raising Responsible Children.* New York: Wyden.
13. Freud, S. (1952). *Interpretation of Dreams.* In *Great Books of the Western World* (vol. 54, Hutchins, R. M., ed.). Chicago: Encyclopedia Britannica.
14. Berne, E., personal communication.
15. Masterson, J. F. (1988). *The Search for the Real Self.* New York: Free Press. Masterson, J. F. (1985) *The Real Self: A Developmental, Self, and Object Relations Approach.* New York: Bruner Mazel.
16. Bartusiak, M. (1988). Cosmic strings. *Discover,* April. Holt, J. (2006). Unstrung. *The New Yorker,* October 2.
17. Frank, J. D. (1974). *Persuasion and Healing.* New York: Schoken Books.
18. Menninger, K. A. (1987). Hope. *Bulletin. Menninger Clinic* 51. Also comment made at Grand Rounds, University of California, Los Angeles, Neuropsychiatric Institute.
19. May, R. (1969). *Love and Will.* New York: W. W. Norton.
20. Boldrini, M., Giovanni, P. A., et al. (1998). Applications of chaos theories to psychiatry. *CNS Spectrums* 3 (January). Petree , J. (2002). Chaos index. www.wfu.edu/petreejh.
21. http://en.wikipedia.org/wiki/butterflyeffect
22. http://en.wikipedia.org/wiki/Attractor
23. Von Foerster, H. (1973, 2003). On constructing a reality. Reprinted in *Understanding Understanding: Essays on Cybernetics and Cognition* (vol.2, Von Foerster, H., ed.). New York: Springer.

Chapter 8

1. Gaylin, W. (1984). *The Rage Within: Anger in Modern Life.* New York: Simon and Schuster.

2. Fairbairn, W. R. D. (1952). *Psychoanalytic Studies of the Personality.* London: RKP.
3. Maciejewski, P. K., Zhang, B., Block, S. D., and Prigerson, H. G. (2007). An empirical examination of the stage theory of grief. *JAMA* 29 (February 21).
4. Masterson, J. (1976). *Psychotherapy of the Borderline Adult: A Developmental Approach.* New York: Brunner Mazel.
5. Karasu, T. B., and Bellak, L. (eds.). (1980). *Specialized Techniques in Individual Therapy.* New York: Bruner Mazel.

Chapter 9

1. Mitscherlich, A., and Mielke, F. (1949). *Doctors of Infamy: The Story of Medical Crimes.* New York: H. Schuyman.
2. Lifton, R. J. (1986). *The Nazi Doctors: Medical Killing and the Psychology of Genocide.* New York: Basic Books.
3. Goethe von, J. W. www.Quotationsbook.com
4. Arendt, H. (1963). *Eichmann in Jerusalem.* New York: Penguin Books.
5. Osler, W. (1985). *Counsels and Ideals and Selected Aphorisms.* Birmingham, AL: Classics of Medicine Library.
6. Erickson, M. H., and Rosen, S. (eds.). (1991). *My Voice Will Go with You: The Teaching Tales of Milton H. Erickson, M.D.* New York: W. W. Norton

INDEX

ABOUT THE AUTHORS

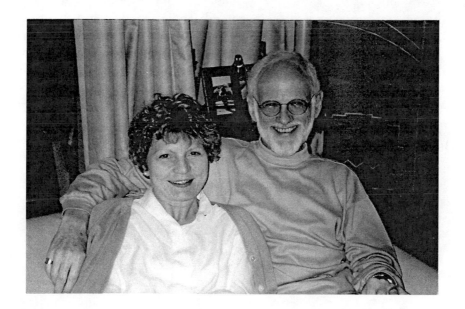

Sheldon H. Kardener, MD graduated with a Bachelor of Science in mechanical engineering and subsequently a doctorate from the School of Medicine, with honors, Alpha Omega Alpha, at Wayne State University. After completing a psychiatric residency at the University of California at Los Angeles, he joined the faculty where he is now a Clinical Professor of Psychiatry. He has been a Fellow of the American Psychiatric Association, Fellow of the American Society of Clinical Hypnosis, and is Board Certified in Psychiatry and Neurology. For over forty years, he has written extensively, practiced psychodynamic psychotherapy—with a special interest in couples therapy—taught mental health professionals, psychiatrists, psychologists, social workers, marriage family therapists, and nurses, as well as lay groups, in the United States and Europe. In the book, *Breaking Free,* he distills these experiences, illuminating his unique approach to understanding how emotional conflicts develop and are treated in psychotherapy.

Monika Olofsson Kardener, MFT was born and raised on the enchanting Swedish island of Gotland. She lived and worked in Germany and England before coming to the United States where she graduated from the University of California at Los Angeles, summa cum laude, Phi Beta Kappa. Subsequently she obtained a master's degree in Islamic studies at UCLA, and a master's degree in psychology from Pepperdine University. She practices as a licensed marriage and family therapist in California. Drawing from her rich and varied background and experiences, she contributes valuable perspectives as co-author of the book, *Breaking Free: How Chains From Childhood Keep Us From What We Want.* In addition to her psychotherapy activities, she is a fine artist specializing in pastels.

Dr. and Mrs. Kardener maintain an office in Santa Monica and a summer home on Gotland.

BUY A SHARE OF THE FUTURE IN YOUR COMMUNITY

These certificates make great holiday, graduation and birthday gifts that can be personalized with the recipient's name. The cost of one S.H.A.R.E. or one square foot is $54.17. The personalized certificate is suitable for framing and will state the number of shares purchased and the amount of each share, as well as the recipient's name. The home that you participate in "building" will last for many years and will continue to grow in value.

Here is a sample SHARE certificate:

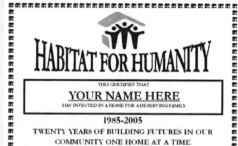

HABITAT FOR HUMANITY

THIS CERTIFIES THAT
YOUR NAME HERE
HAS INVESTED IN A HOME FOR A DESERVING FAMILY

1985-2005
TWENTY YEARS OF BUILDING FUTURES IN OUR
COMMUNITY ONE HOME AT A TIME

1200 SQUARE FOOT HOUSE @ $65,000 = $54.17 PER SQUARE FOOT
This certificate represents a tax deductible donation. It has no cash value.

YES, I WOULD LIKE TO HELP!

I support the work that Habitat for Humanity does and I want to be part of the excitement! As a donor, I will receive periodic updates on your construction activities but, more importantly, I know my gift will help a family in our community realize the dream of homeownership. **I would like to SHARE in your efforts against substandard housing in my community!** *(Please print below)*

PLEASE SEND ME _____ SHARES at $54.17 EACH = $ $_____

In Honor Of: _____

Occasion: (Circle One)   HOLIDAY   BIRTHDAY   ANNIVERSARY

         OTHER: _____

Address of Recipient: _____

Gift From: _____ *Donor Address:* _____

Donor Email: _____

I AM ENCLOSING A CHECK FOR $ $_____ PAYABLE TO HABITAT FOR HUMANITY OR PLEASE CHARGE MY VISA OR MASTERCARD *(CIRCLE ONE)*

Card Number _____ Expiration Date: _____

Name as it appears on Credit Card _____ Charge Amount $ _____

Signature _____

Billing Address _____

Telephone # Day _____ Eve _____

PLEASE NOTE: Your contribution is tax-deductible to the fullest extent allowed by law.
Habitat for Humanity • P.O. Box 1443 • Newport News, VA 23601 • 757-596-5553
www.HelpHabitatforHumanity.org

LaVergne, TN USA
01 December 2009
165706LV00001B/162/P